50% OFF Kaplan Nu
School Entrance Exam Course!

By Mometrix

Dear Customer,

We consider it an honor and a privilege that you chose our Kaplan Nursing School Entrance Exam Study Guide. As a way of showing our appreciation and to help us better serve you, we are offering **50% off our online Kaplan Nursing School Entrance Exam Prep Course.** Many Kaplan Entrance Exam courses are needlessly expensive and don't deliver enough value. With our course, you get access to the best Kaplan Nursing School Entrance Exam prep material, and **you only pay half price**.

We have structured our online course to perfectly complement your printed study guide. The Kaplan Entrance Exam Online Course contains **in-depth lessons** that cover all the most important topics, **180+ video reviews** that explain difficult concepts, over **600 practice questions** to ensure you feel prepared, and more than 250 digital flashcards, so you can study while you're on the go.

Online Kaplan Nursing School Entrance Exam Prep Course

Topics Included:

- Reading Comprehension
    - Common Organizations of Texts
    - Reading Argumentative Writing
- Reading Argumentative Writing Reading Comprehension
    - Common Organizations of Texts
    - Reading Argumentative Writing
- Writing
    - The Writing Process
    - Outlining and Organizing Ideas
- Mathematics
    - Operations
    - Properties of Exponents
- Science
    - Scientific Inquiry and Reasoning
    - Cell Cycle and Cellular Division

Course Features:

- Kaplan Nursing School Entrance Exam Study Guide
    - Get content that complements our best-selling study guide.
- Full-Length Practice Tests
    - With over 600 practice questions, you can test yourself again and again.
- Mobile Friendly
    - If you need to study on the go, the course is easily accessible from your mobile device.
- Kaplan Nursing School Exam Flashcards
    - Our course includes a flashcard mode with over 250 content cards to help you study.

To receive this discount, visit us at mometrix.com/university/kaplan or simply scan this QR code with your smartphone. At the checkout page, enter the discount code: **kap50off**

If you have any questions or concerns, please contact us at support@mometrix.com.

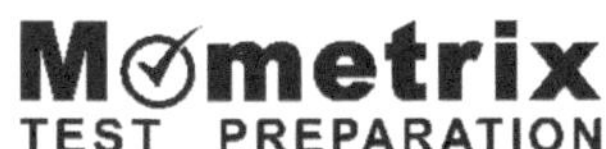

FREE Study Skills Videos/DVD Offer

Dear Customer,

Thank you for your purchase from Mometrix! We consider it an honor and a privilege that you have purchased our product and we want to ensure your satisfaction.

As part of our ongoing effort to meet the needs of test takers, we have developed a set of Study Skills Videos that we would like to give you for FREE. These videos cover our *best practices* for getting ready for your exam, from how to use our study materials to how to best prepare for the day of the test.

All that we ask is that you email us with feedback that would describe your experience so far with our product. Good, bad, or indifferent, we want to know what you think!

To get your FREE Study Skills Videos, you can use the **QR code** below, or send us an **email** at studyvideos@mometrix.com with *FREE VIDEOS* in the subject line and the following information in the body of the email:

- The name of the product you purchased.
- Your product rating on a scale of 1-5, with 5 being the highest rating.
- Your feedback. It can be long, short, or anything in between. We just want to know your impressions and experience so far with our product. (Good feedback might include how our study material met your needs and ways we might be able to make it even better. You could highlight features that you found helpful or features that you think we should add.)

If you have any questions or concerns, please don't hesitate to contact me directly.

Thanks again!

Sincerely,

Jay Willis
Vice President
jay.willis@mometrix.com
1-800-673-8175

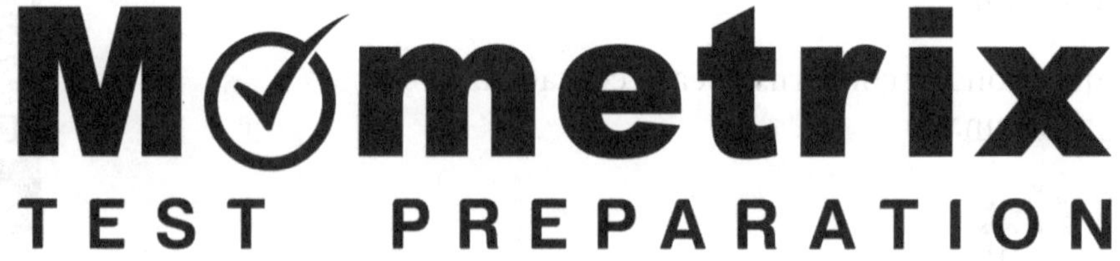

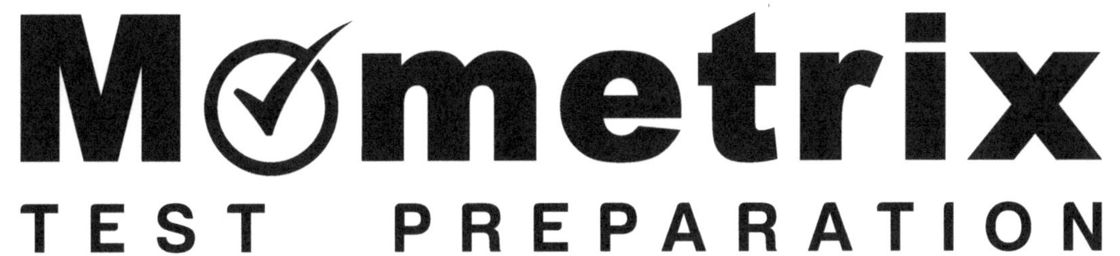

Kaplan Nursing School Entrance Exam Prep 2025-2026

Secrets Study Guide with Detailed Answer Explanations

3 Full-Length Practice Tests

150+ Online Video Tutorials

5th Edition

Written and edited by Matthew Bowling

Printed in the United States of America

This paper meets the requirements of ANSI/NISO Z39.48-1992 (Permanence of Paper).

ISBN 13: 978-1-5167-2737-7
ISBN 10: 1-5167-2737-1

DEAR FUTURE EXAM SUCCESS STORY

First of all, **THANK YOU** for purchasing Mometrix study materials!

Second, congratulations! You are one of the few determined test-takers who are committed to doing whatever it takes to excel on your exam. **You have come to the right place.** We developed these study materials with one goal in mind: to deliver you the information you need in a format that's concise and easy to use.

In addition to optimizing your guide for the content of the test, we've outlined our recommended steps for breaking down the preparation process into small, attainable goals so you can make sure you stay on track.

We've also analyzed the entire test-taking process, identifying the most common pitfalls and showing how you can overcome them and be ready for any curveball the test throws you.

Standardized testing is one of the biggest obstacles on your road to success, which only increases the importance of doing well in the high-pressure, high-stakes environment of test day. Your results on this test could have a significant impact on your future, and this guide provides the information and practical advice to help you achieve your full potential on test day.

Your success is our success

We would love to hear from you! If you would like to share the story of your exam success or if you have any questions or comments in regard to our products, please contact us at **800-673-8175** or **support@mometrix.com**.

Thanks again for your business and we wish you continued success!

Sincerely,
The Mometrix Test Preparation Team

TABLE OF CONTENTS

Introduction

Thank you for purchasing this resource! You have made the choice to prepare yourself for a test that could have a huge impact on your future, and this guide is designed to help you be fully ready for test day. Obviously, it's important to have a solid understanding of the test material, but you also need to be prepared for the unique environment and stressors of the test, so that you can perform to the best of your abilities.

For this purpose, the first section that appears in this guide is the **Secret Keys**. We've devoted countless hours to meticulously researching what works and what doesn't, and we've boiled down our findings to the five most impactful steps you can take to improve your performance on the test. We start at the beginning with study planning and move through the preparation process, all the way to the testing strategies that will help you get the most out of what you know when you're finally sitting in front of the test.

We recommend that you start preparing for your test as far in advance as possible. However, if you've bought this guide as a last-minute study resource and only have a few days before your test, we recommend that you skip over the first two Secret Keys since they address a long-term study plan.

If you struggle with **test anxiety**, we strongly encourage you to check out our recommendations for how you can overcome it. Test anxiety is a formidable foe, but it can be beaten, and we want to make sure you have the tools you need to defeat it.

Review Video Directory

As you work your way through this guide, you will see numerous review video links interspersed with the written content. If you would like to access all of these review videos in one place, click on the video directory link found on the bonus page: **mometrix.com/bonus948/kaplannursing**

Secret Key #1 – Plan Big, Study Small

There's a lot riding on your performance. If you want to ace this test, you're going to need to keep your skills sharp and the material fresh in your mind. You need a plan that lets you review everything you need to know while still fitting in your schedule. We'll break this strategy down into three categories.

Information Organization

Start with the information you already have: the official test outline. From this, you can make a complete list of all the concepts you need to cover before the test. Organize these concepts into groups that can be studied together, and create a list of any related vocabulary you need to learn so you can brush up on any difficult terms. You'll want to keep this vocabulary list handy once you actually start studying since you may need to add to it along the way.

Time Management

Once you have your set of study concepts, decide how to spread them out over the time you have left before the test. Break your study plan into small, clear goals so you have a manageable task for each day and know exactly what you're doing. Then just focus on one small step at a time. When you manage your time this way, you don't need to spend hours at a time studying. Studying a small block of content for a short period each day helps you retain information better and avoid stressing over how much you have left to do. You can relax knowing that you have a plan to cover everything in time. In order for this strategy to be effective though, you have to start studying early and stick to your schedule. Avoid the exhaustion and futility that comes from last-minute cramming!

Study Environment

The environment you study in has a big impact on your learning. Studying in a coffee shop, while probably more enjoyable, is not likely to be as fruitful as studying in a quiet room. It's important to keep distractions to a minimum. You're only planning to study for a short block of time, so make the most of it. Don't pause to check your phone or get up to find a snack. It's also important to **avoid multitasking**. Research has consistently shown that multitasking will make your studying dramatically less effective. Your study area should also be comfortable and well-lit so you don't have the distraction of straining your eyes or sitting on an uncomfortable chair.

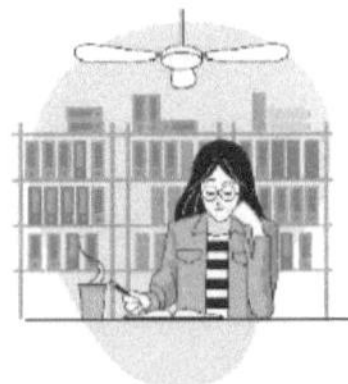

The time of day you study is also important. You want to be rested and alert. Don't wait until just before bedtime. Study when you'll be most likely to comprehend and remember. Even better, if you know what time of day your test will be, set that time aside for study. That way your brain will be used to working on that subject at that specific time and you'll have a better chance of recalling information.

Finally, it can be helpful to team up with others who are studying for the same test. Your actual studying should be done in as isolated an environment as possible, but the work of organizing the information and setting up the study plan can be divided up. In between study sessions, you can discuss with your teammates the concepts that you're all studying and quiz each other on the details. Just be sure that your teammates are as serious about the test as you are. If you find that your study time is being replaced with social time, you might need to find a new team.

Secret Key #2 – Make Your Studying Count

You're devoting a lot of time and effort to preparing for this test, so you want to be absolutely certain it will pay off. This means doing more than just reading the content and hoping you can remember it on test day. It's important to make every minute of study count. There are two main areas you can focus on to make your studying count.

Retention

It doesn't matter how much time you study if you can't remember the material. You need to make sure you are retaining the concepts. To check your retention of the information you're learning, try recalling it at later times with minimal prompting. Try carrying around flashcards and glance at one or two from time to time or ask a friend who's also studying for the test to quiz you.

To enhance your retention, look for ways to put the information into practice so that you can apply it rather than simply recalling it. If you're using the information in practical ways, it will be much easier to remember. Similarly, it helps to solidify a concept in your mind if you're not only reading it to yourself but also explaining it to someone else. Ask a friend to let you teach them about a concept you're a little shaky on (or speak aloud to an imaginary audience if necessary). As you try to summarize, define, give examples, and answer your friend's questions, you'll understand the concepts better and they will stay with you longer. Finally, step back for a big picture view and ask yourself how each piece of information fits with the whole subject. When you link the different concepts together and see them working together as a whole, it's easier to remember the individual components.

Finally, practice showing your work on any multi-step problems, even if you're just studying. Writing out each step you take to solve a problem will help solidify the process in your mind, and you'll be more likely to remember it during the test.

Modality

Modality simply refers to the means or method by which you study. Choosing a study modality that fits your own individual learning style is crucial. No two people learn best in exactly the same way, so it's important to know your strengths and use them to your advantage.

For example, if you learn best by visualization, focus on visualizing a concept in your mind and draw an image or a diagram. Try color-coding your notes, illustrating them, or creating symbols that will trigger your mind to recall a learned concept. If you learn best by hearing or discussing information, find a study partner who learns the same way or read aloud to yourself. Think about how to put the information in your own words. Imagine that you are giving a lecture on the topic and record yourself so you can listen to it later.

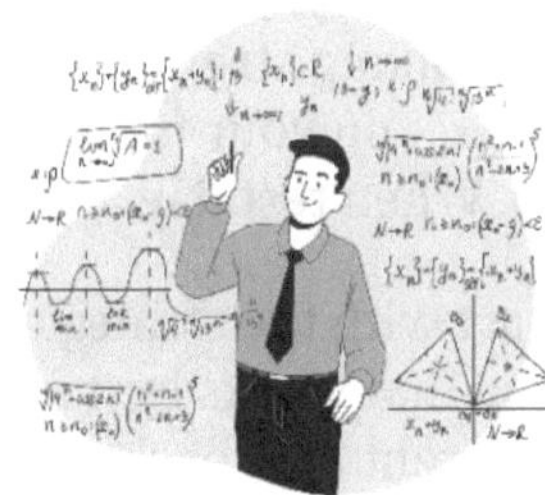

For any learning style, flashcards can be helpful. Organize the information so you can take advantage of spare moments to review. Underline key words or phrases. Use different colors for different categories. Mnemonic devices (such as creating a short list in which every item starts with the same letter) can also help with retention. Find what works best for you and use it to store the information in your mind most effectively and easily.

Secret Key #3 – Practice the Right Way

Your success on test day depends not only on how many hours you put into preparing, but also on whether you prepared the right way. It's good to check along the way to see if your studying is paying off. One of the most effective ways to do this is by taking practice tests to evaluate your progress. Practice tests are useful because they show exactly where you need to improve. Every time you take a practice test, pay special attention to these three groups of questions:

- The questions you got wrong
- The questions you had to guess on, even if you guessed right
- The questions you found difficult or slow to work through

This will show you exactly what your weak areas are, and where you need to devote more study time. Ask yourself why each of these questions gave you trouble. Was it because you didn't understand the material? Was it because you didn't remember the vocabulary? Do you need more repetitions on this type of question to build speed and confidence? Dig into those questions and figure out how you can strengthen your weak areas as you go back to review the material.

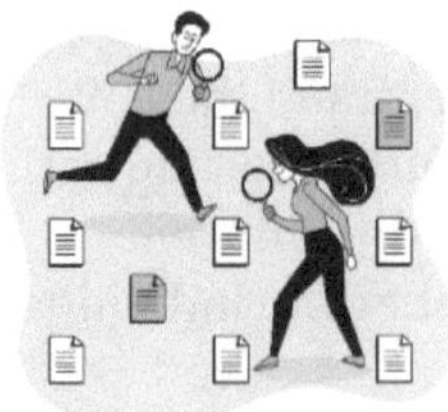

Additionally, many practice tests have a section explaining the answer choices. It can be tempting to read the explanation and think that you now have a good understanding of the concept. However, an explanation likely only covers part of the question's broader context. Even if the explanation makes perfect sense, **go back and investigate** every concept related to the question until you're positive you have a thorough understanding.

As you go along, keep in mind that the practice test is just that: practice. Memorizing these questions and answers will not be very helpful on the actual test because it is unlikely to have any of the same exact questions. If you only know the right answers to the sample questions, you won't be prepared for the real thing. **Study the concepts** until you understand them fully, and then you'll be able to answer any question that shows up on the test.

It's important to wait on the practice tests until you're ready. If you take a test on your first day of study, you may be overwhelmed by the amount of material covered and how much you need to learn. Work up to it gradually.

On test day, you'll need to be prepared for answering questions, managing your time, and using the test-taking strategies you've learned. It's a lot to balance, like a mental marathon that will have a big impact on your future. Like training for a marathon, you'll need to start slowly and work your way up. When test day arrives, you'll be ready.

Start with the strategies you've read in the first two Secret Keys—plan your course and study in the way that works best for you. If you have time, consider using multiple study resources to get different approaches to the same concepts. It can be helpful to see difficult concepts from more than one angle. Then find a good source for practice tests. Many times, the test website will suggest potential study resources or provide sample tests.

Practice Test Strategy

If you're able to find at least three practice tests, we recommend this strategy:

Untimed and Open-Book Practice

Take the first test with no time constraints and with your notes and study guide handy. Take your time and focus on applying the strategies you've learned.

Timed and Open-Book Practice

Take the second practice test open-book as well, but set a timer and practice pacing yourself to finish in time.

Timed and Closed-Book Practice

Take any other practice tests as if it were test day. Set a timer and put away your study materials. Sit at a table or desk in a quiet room, imagine yourself at the testing center, and answer questions as quickly and accurately as possible.

Keep repeating timed and closed-book tests on a regular basis until you run out of practice tests or it's time for the actual test. Your mind will be ready for the schedule and stress of test day, and you'll be able to focus on recalling the material you've learned.

Secret Key #4 – Pace Yourself

Once you're fully prepared for the material on the test, your biggest challenge on test day will be managing your time. Just knowing that the clock is ticking can make you panic even if you have plenty of time left. Work on pacing yourself so you can build confidence against the time constraints of the exam. Pacing is a difficult skill to master, especially in a high-pressure environment, so **practice is vital**.

Set time expectations for your pace based on how much time is available. For example, if a section has 60 questions and the time limit is 30 minutes, you know you have to average 30 seconds or less per question in order to answer them all. Although 30 seconds is the hard limit, set 25 seconds per question as your goal, so you reserve extra time to spend on harder questions. When you budget extra time for the harder questions, you no longer have any reason to stress when those questions take longer to answer.

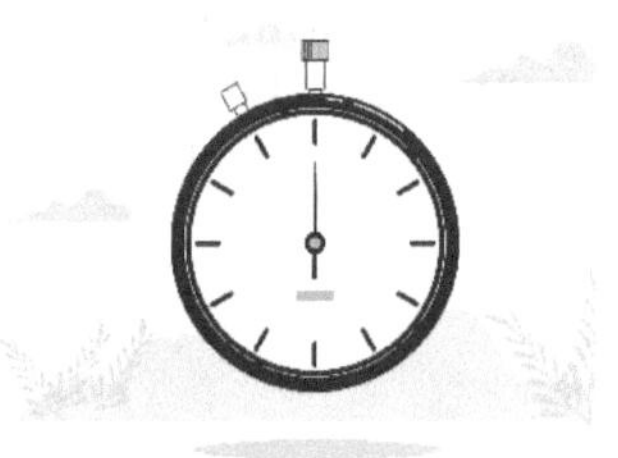

Don't let this time expectation distract you from working through the test at a calm, steady pace, but keep it in mind so you don't spend too much time on any one question. Recognize that taking extra time on one question you don't understand may keep you from answering two that you do understand later in the test. If your time limit for a question is up and you're still not sure of the answer, mark it and move on, and come back to it later if the time and the test format allow. If the testing format doesn't allow you to return to earlier questions, just make an educated guess; then put it out of your mind and move on.

On the easier questions, be careful not to rush. It may seem wise to hurry through them so you have more time for the challenging ones, but it's not worth missing one if you know the concept and just didn't take the time to read the question fully. Work efficiently but make sure you understand the question and have looked at all of the answer choices, since more than one may seem right at first.

Even if you're paying attention to the time, you may find yourself a little behind at some point. You should speed up to get back on track, but do so wisely. Don't panic; just take a few seconds less on each question until you're caught up. Don't guess without thinking, but do look through the answer choices and eliminate any you know are wrong. If you can get down to two choices, it is often worthwhile to guess from those. Once you've chosen an answer, move on and don't dwell on any that you skipped or had to hurry through. If a question was taking too long, chances are it was one of the harder ones, so you weren't as likely to get it right anyway.

On the other hand, if you find yourself getting ahead of schedule, it may be beneficial to slow down a little. The more quickly you work, the more likely you are to make a careless mistake that will affect your score. You've budgeted time for each question, so don't be afraid to spend that time. Practice an efficient but careful pace to get the most out of the time you have.

Secret Key #5 – Have a Plan for Guessing

When you're taking the test, you may find yourself stuck on a question. Some of the answer choices seem better than others, but you don't see the one answer choice that is obviously correct. What do you do?

The scenario described above is very common, yet most test takers have not effectively prepared for it. Developing and practicing a plan for guessing may be one of the single most effective uses of your time as you get ready for the exam.

In developing your plan for guessing, there are three questions to address:

- When should you start the guessing process?
- How should you narrow down the choices?
- Which answer should you choose?

When to Start the Guessing Process

Unless your plan for guessing is to select C every time (which, despite its merits, is not what we recommend), you need to leave yourself enough time to apply your answer elimination strategies. Since you have a limited amount of time for each question, that means that if you're going to give yourself the best shot at guessing correctly, you have to decide quickly whether or not you will guess.

Of course, the best-case scenario is that you don't have to guess at all, so first, see if you can answer the question based on your knowledge of the subject and basic reasoning skills. Focus on the key words in the question and try to jog your memory of related topics. Give yourself a chance to bring the knowledge to mind, but once you realize that you don't have (or you can't access) the knowledge you need to answer the question, it's time to start the guessing process.

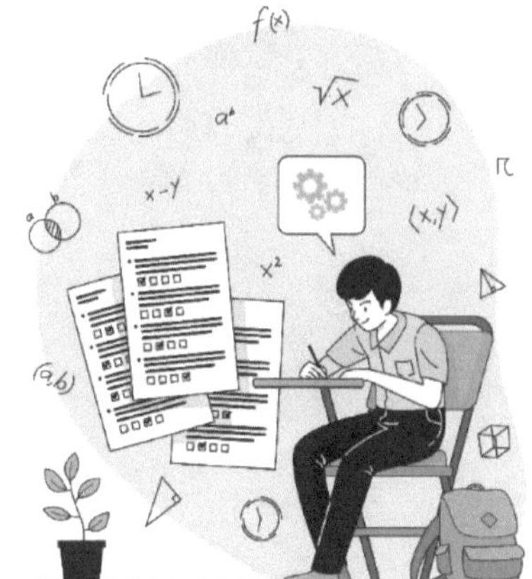

It's almost always better to start the guessing process too early than too late. It only takes a few seconds to remember something and answer the question from knowledge. Carefully eliminating wrong answer choices takes longer. Plus, going through the process of eliminating answer choices can actually help jog your memory.

Summary: Start the guessing process as soon as you decide that you can't answer the question based on your knowledge.

How to Narrow Down the Choices

The next chapter in this book (**Test-Taking Strategies**) includes a wide range of strategies for how to approach questions and how to look for answer choices to eliminate. You will definitely want to read those carefully, practice them, and figure out which ones work best for you. Here though, we're going to address a mindset rather than a particular strategy.

Your odds of guessing an answer correctly depend on how many options you are choosing from.

Number of options left	5	4	3	2	1
Odds of guessing correctly	20%	25%	33%	50%	100%

You can see from this chart just how valuable it is to be able to eliminate incorrect answers and make an educated guess, but there are two things that many test takers do that cause them to miss out on the benefits of guessing:

- Accidentally eliminating the correct answer
- Selecting an answer based on an impression

We'll look at the first one here, and the second one in the next section.

To avoid accidentally eliminating the correct answer, we recommend a thought exercise called **the $5 challenge**. In this challenge, you only eliminate an answer choice from contention if you are willing to bet $5 on it being wrong. Why $5? Five dollars is a small but not insignificant amount of money. It's an amount you could afford to lose but wouldn't want to throw away. And while losing $5 once might not hurt too much, doing it twenty times will set you back $100. In the same way, each small decision you make—eliminating a choice here, guessing on a question there—won't by itself impact your score very much, but when you put them all together, they can make a big difference. By holding each answer choice elimination decision to a higher standard, you can reduce the risk of accidentally eliminating the correct answer.

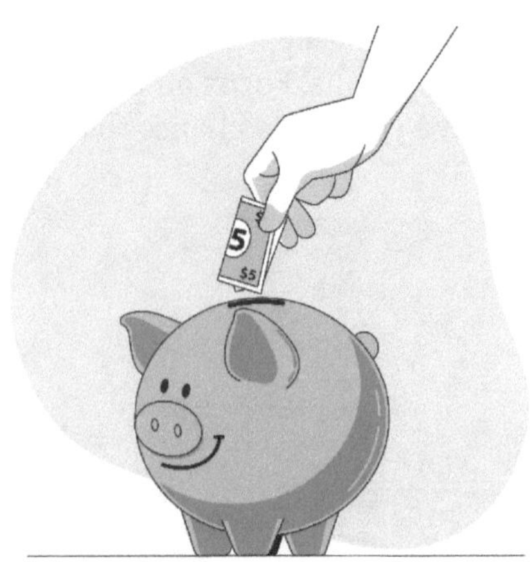

The $5 challenge can also be applied in a positive sense: If you are willing to bet $5 that an answer choice *is* correct, go ahead and mark it as correct.

Summary: Only eliminate an answer choice if you are willing to bet $5 that it is wrong.

Which Answer to Choose

You're taking the test. You've run into a hard question and decided you'll have to guess. You've eliminated all the answer choices you're willing to bet $5 on. Now you have to pick an answer. Why do we even need to talk about this? Why can't you just pick whichever one you feel like when the time comes?

The answer to these questions is that if you don't come into the test with a plan, you'll rely on your impression to select an answer choice, and if you do that, you risk falling into a trap. The test writers know that everyone who takes their test will be guessing on some of the questions, so they intentionally write wrong answer choices to seem plausible. You still have to pick an answer though, and if the wrong answer choices are designed to look right, how can you ever be sure that you're not falling for their trap? The best solution we've found to this dilemma is to take the decision out of your hands entirely. Here is the process we recommend:

Once you've eliminated any choices that you are confident (willing to bet $5) are wrong, select the first remaining choice as your answer.

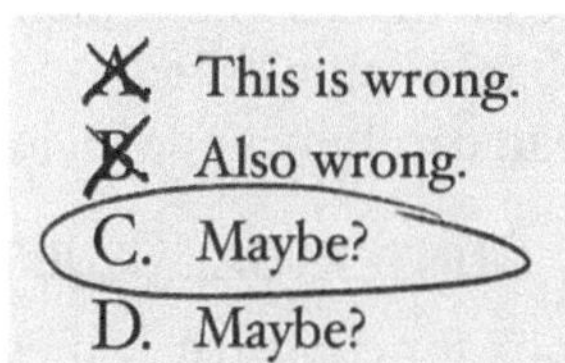

Whether you choose to select the first remaining choice, the second, or the last, the important thing is that you use some preselected standard. Using this approach guarantees that you will not be enticed into selecting an answer choice that looks right, because you are not basing your decision on how the answer choices look.

This is not meant to make you question your knowledge. Instead, it is to help you recognize the difference between your knowledge and your impressions. There's a huge difference between thinking an answer is right because of what you know, and thinking an answer is right because it looks or sounds like it should be right.

Summary: To ensure that your selection is appropriately random, make a predetermined selection from among all answer choices you have not eliminated.

Test-Taking Strategies

This section contains a list of test-taking strategies that you may find helpful as you work through the test. By taking what you know and applying logical thought, you can maximize your chances of answering any question correctly!

It is very important to realize that every question is different and every person is different: no single strategy will work on every question, and no single strategy will work for every person. That's why we've included all of them here, so you can try them out and determine which ones work best for different types of questions and which ones work best for you.

Question Strategies

⊘ Read Carefully

Read the question and the answer choices carefully. Don't miss the question because you misread the terms. You have plenty of time to read each question thoroughly and make sure you understand what is being asked. Yet a happy medium must be attained, so don't waste too much time. You must read carefully and efficiently.

⊘ Contextual Clues

Look for contextual clues. If the question includes a word you are not familiar with, look at the immediate context for some indication of what the word might mean. Contextual clues can often give you all the information you need to decipher the meaning of an unfamiliar word. Even if you can't determine the meaning, you may be able to narrow down the possibilities enough to make a solid guess at the answer to the question.

⊘ Prefixes

If you're having trouble with a word in the question or answer choices, try dissecting it. Take advantage of every clue that the word might include. Prefixes can be a huge help. Usually, they allow you to determine a basic meaning. *Pre-* means before, *post-* means after, *pro-* is positive, *de-* is negative. From prefixes, you can get an idea of the general meaning of the word and try to put it into context.

⊘ Hedge Words

Watch out for critical hedge words, such as *likely*, *may*, *can*, *sometimes*, *often*, *almost*, *mostly*, *usually*, *generally*, *rarely*, and *sometimes*. Question writers insert these hedge phrases to cover every possibility. Often an answer choice will be wrong simply because it leaves no room for exception. Be on guard for answer choices that have definitive words such as *exactly* and *always*.

⊘ Switchback Words

Stay alert for *switchbacks*. These are the words and phrases frequently used to alert you to shifts in thought. The most common switchback words are *but*, *although*, and *however*. Others include *nevertheless*, *on the other hand*, *even though*, *while*, *in spite of*, *despite*, and *regardless of*. Switchback words are important to catch because they can change the direction of the question or an answer choice.

☑ Face Value

When in doubt, use common sense. Accept the situation in the problem at face value. Don't read too much into it. These problems will not require you to make wild assumptions. If you have to go beyond creativity and warp time or space in order to have an answer choice fit the question, then you should move on and consider the other answer choices. These are normal problems rooted in reality. The applicable relationship or explanation may not be readily apparent, but it is there for you to figure out. Use your common sense to interpret anything that isn't clear.

Answer Choice Strategies

☑ Answer Selection

The most thorough way to pick an answer choice is to identify and eliminate wrong answers until only one is left, then confirm it is the correct answer. Sometimes an answer choice may immediately seem right, but be careful. The test writers will usually put more than one reasonable answer choice on each question, so take a second to read all of them and make sure that the other choices are not equally obvious. As long as you have time left, it is better to read every answer choice than to pick the first one that looks right without checking the others.

☑ Answer Choice Families

An answer choice family consists of two (in rare cases, three) answer choices that are very similar in construction and cannot all be true at the same time. If you see two answer choices that are direct opposites or parallels, one of them is usually the correct answer. For instance, if one answer choice says that quantity x increases and another either says that quantity x decreases (opposite) or says that quantity y increases (parallel), then those answer choices would fall into the same family. An answer choice that doesn't match the construction of the answer choice family is more likely to be incorrect. Most questions will not have answer choice families, but when they do appear, you should be prepared to recognize them.

☑ Eliminate Answers

Eliminate answer choices as soon as you realize they are wrong, but make sure you consider all possibilities. If you are eliminating answer choices and realize that the last one you are left with is also wrong, don't panic. Start over and consider each choice again. There may be something you missed the first time that you will realize on the second pass.

☑ Avoid Fact Traps

Don't be distracted by an answer choice that is factually true but doesn't answer the question. You are looking for the choice that answers the question. Stay focused on what the question is asking for so you don't accidentally pick an answer that is true but incorrect. Always go back to the question and make sure the answer choice you've selected actually answers the question and is not merely a true statement.

☑ Extreme Statements

In general, you should avoid answers that put forth extreme actions as standard practice or proclaim controversial ideas as established fact. An answer choice that states the "process should be used in certain situations, if..." is much more likely to be correct than one that states the "process should be discontinued completely." The first is a calm rational statement and doesn't even make a definitive, uncompromising stance, using a hedge word *if* to provide wiggle room, whereas the second choice is far more extreme.

✓ Benchmark

As you read through the answer choices and you come across one that seems to answer the question well, mentally select that answer choice. This is not your final answer, but it's the one that will help you evaluate the other answer choices. The one that you selected is your benchmark or standard for judging each of the other answer choices. Every other answer choice must be compared to your benchmark. That choice is correct until proven otherwise by another answer choice beating it. If you find a better answer, then that one becomes your new benchmark. Once you've decided that no other choice answers the question as well as your benchmark, you have your final answer.

✓ Predict the Answer

Before you even start looking at the answer choices, it is often best to try to predict the answer. When you come up with the answer on your own, it is easier to avoid distractions and traps because you will know exactly what to look for. The right answer choice is unlikely to be word-for-word what you came up with, but it should be a close match. Even if you are confident that you have the right answer, you should still take the time to read each option before moving on.

General Strategies

✓ Tough Questions

If you are stumped on a problem or it appears too hard or too difficult, don't waste time. Move on! Remember though, if you can quickly check for obviously incorrect answer choices, your chances of guessing correctly are greatly improved. Before you completely give up, at least try to knock out a couple of possible answers. Eliminate what you can and then guess at the remaining answer choices before moving on.

✓ Check Your Work

Since you will probably not know every term listed and the answer to every question, it is important that you get credit for the ones that you do know. Don't miss any questions through careless mistakes. If at all possible, try to take a second to look back over your answer selection and make sure you've selected the correct answer choice and haven't made a costly careless mistake (such as marking an answer choice that you didn't mean to mark). This quick double check should more than pay for itself in caught mistakes for the time it costs.

✓ Pace Yourself

It's easy to be overwhelmed when you're looking at a page full of questions; your mind is confused and full of random thoughts, and the clock is ticking down faster than you would like. Calm down and maintain the pace that you have set for yourself. Especially as you get down to the last few minutes of the test, don't let the small numbers on the clock make you panic. As long as you are on track by monitoring your pace, you are guaranteed to have time for each question.

✓ Don't Rush

It is very easy to make errors when you are in a hurry. Maintaining a fast pace in answering questions is pointless if it makes you miss questions that you would have gotten right otherwise. Test writers like to include distracting information and wrong answers that seem right. Taking a little extra time to avoid careless mistakes can make all the difference in your test score. Find a pace that allows you to be confident in the answers that you select.

✓ KEEP MOVING

Panicking will not help you pass the test, so do your best to stay calm and keep moving. Taking deep breaths and going through the answer elimination steps you practiced can help to break through a stress barrier and keep your pace.

Final Notes

The combination of a solid foundation of content knowledge and the confidence that comes from practicing your plan for applying that knowledge is the key to maximizing your performance on test day. As your foundation of content knowledge is built up and strengthened, you'll find that the strategies included in this chapter become more and more effective in helping you quickly sift through the distractions and traps of the test to isolate the correct answer.

Now that you're preparing to move forward into the test content chapters of this book, be sure to keep your goal in mind. As you read, think about how you will be able to apply this information on the test. If you've already seen sample questions for the test and you have an idea of the question format and style, try to come up with questions of your own that you can answer based on what you're reading. This will give you valuable practice applying your knowledge in the same ways you can expect to on test day.

Good luck and good studying!

Reading Comprehension

Transform passive reading into active learning! After immersing yourself in this chapter, put your comprehension to the test by taking a quiz. The insights you gained will stay with you longer this way. Scan the QR code to go directly to the chapter quiz interface for this study guide. If you're using a computer, simply visit the bonus page at **mometrix.com/bonus948/kaplannursing** and click the Chapter Quizzes link.

Main Ideas and Supporting Details

Identifying Topics and Main Ideas

One of the most important skills in reading comprehension is the identification of **topics** and **main ideas**. There is a subtle difference between these two features. The topic is the subject of a text (i.e., what the text is all about). The main idea, on the other hand, is the most important point being made by the author. The topic is usually expressed in a few words at the most while the main idea often needs a full sentence to be completely defined. As an example, a short passage might be written on the topic of penguins, and the main idea could be written as *Penguins are different from other birds in many ways*. In most nonfiction writing, the topic and the main idea will be **stated directly** and often appear in a sentence at the very beginning or end of the text. When being tested on an understanding of the author's topic, you may be able to skim the passage for the general idea by reading only the first sentence of each paragraph. A body paragraph's first sentence is often—but not always—the main **topic sentence** which gives you a summary of the content in the paragraph.

However, there are cases in which the reader must figure out an **unstated** topic or main idea. In these instances, you must read every sentence of the text and try to come up with an overarching idea that is supported by each of those sentences.

Note: The main idea should not be confused with the thesis statement. While the main idea gives a brief, general summary of a text, the thesis statement provides a **specific perspective** on an issue that the author supports with evidence.

Review Video: Topics and Main Ideas
Visit mometrix.com/academy and enter code: 407801

Supporting Details

Supporting details are smaller pieces of evidence that provide backing for the main point. In order to show that a main idea is correct or valid, an author must add details that prove their point. All texts contain details, but they are only classified as supporting details when they serve to reinforce some larger point. Supporting details are most commonly found in informative and persuasive texts. In some cases, they will be clearly indicated with terms like *for example* or *for instance*, or they will be enumerated with terms like *first*, *second*, and *last*. However, you need to be prepared for texts that do not contain those indicators. As a reader, you should consider whether the author's supporting details really back up his or her main point. Details can be factual and correct, yet they may not be **relevant** to the author's point. Conversely, details can be relevant, but be ineffective because they are based on opinion or assertions that cannot be proven.

> **Review Video: Supporting Details**
> Visit mometrix.com/academy and enter code: 396297

Author's Purpose

Author's Purpose

Usually, identifying the author's **purpose** is easier than identifying his or her **position**. In most cases, the author has no interest in hiding his or her purpose. A text that is meant to entertain, for instance, should be written to please the reader. Most narratives, or stories, are written to entertain, though they may also inform or persuade. Informative texts are easy to identify, while the most difficult purpose of a text to identify is persuasion because the author has an interest in making this purpose hard to detect. When a reader discovers that the author is trying to persuade, he or she should be skeptical of the argument. For this reason, persuasive texts often try to establish an entertaining tone and hope to amuse the reader into agreement. On the other hand, an informative tone may be implemented to create an appearance of authority and objectivity.

An author's purpose is evident often in the **organization** of the text (e.g., section headings in bold font points to an informative text). However, you may not have such organization available to you in your exam. Instead, if the author makes his or her main idea clear from the beginning, then the likely purpose of the text is to **inform**. If the author begins by making a claim and provides various arguments to support that claim, then the purpose is probably to **persuade**. If the author tells a story or wants to gain the reader's attention more than to push a particular point or deliver information, then his or her purpose is most likely to **entertain**. As a reader, you must judge authors on how well they accomplish their purpose. In other words, you need to consider the type of passage (e.g., technical, persuasive, etc.) that the author has written and if the author has followed the requirements of the passage type.

> **Review Video: Understanding the Author's Intent**
> Visit mometrix.com/academy and enter code: 511819

Informational Texts

An **informational text** is written to educate and enlighten readers. Informational texts are almost always nonfiction and are rarely structured as a story. The intention of an informational text is to deliver information in the most comprehensible way. So, look for the structure of the text to be very clear. In an informational text, the thesis statement is one or two sentences that normally appears at the end of the first paragraph. The author may use some colorful language, but he or she is likely to put more emphasis on clarity and precision. Informational essays do not typically appeal to the emotions. They often contain facts and figures and rarely include the opinion of the author; however, readers should remain aware of the possibility for bias as those facts are presented. Sometimes a persuasive essay can resemble an informative essay, especially if the author maintains an even tone and presents his or her views as if they were established fact.

> **Review Video: Informational Text**
> Visit mometrix.com/academy and enter code: 924964

Persuasive Writing

In a persuasive essay, the author is attempting to change the reader's mind or **convince** him or her of something that he or she did not believe previously. There are several identifying characteristics of **persuasive writing**. One is **opinion presented as fact**. When authors attempt to persuade readers, they often present their opinions as if they were fact. Readers must be on guard for statements that sound factual but which cannot be subjected to research, observation, or experiment. Another characteristic of persuasive writing is **emotional language**. An author will often try to play on the emotions of readers by appealing to their sympathy or sense of morality. When an author uses colorful or evocative language with the intent of arousing the reader's passions, then the author may be attempting to persuade. Finally, in many cases, a persuasive text will give an **unfair explanation of opposing positions**, if these positions are mentioned at all.

Entertaining Texts

The success or failure of an author's intent to **entertain** is determined by those who read the author's work. Entertaining texts may be either fiction or nonfiction, and they may describe real or imagined people, places, and events. Entertaining texts are often narratives or poems. A text that is written to entertain is likely to contain **colorful language** that engages the imagination and the emotions. Such writing often features a great deal of figurative language, which typically enlivens the subject matter with images and analogies.

Though an entertaining text is not usually written to persuade or inform, authors may accomplish both of these tasks in their work. An entertaining text may *appeal to the reader's emotions* and cause him or her to think differently about a particular subject. In any case, entertaining texts tend to showcase the personality of the author more than other types of writing.

Descriptive Text

In a sense, almost all writing is descriptive, insofar as an author seeks to describe events, ideas, or people to the reader. Some texts, however, are primarily concerned with **description**. A descriptive text focuses on a particular subject and attempts to depict the subject in a way that will be clear to readers. Descriptive texts contain many adjectives and adverbs (i.e., words that give shades of meaning and create a more detailed mental picture for the reader). A descriptive text fails when it is unclear to the reader. A descriptive text will certainly be informative and may be persuasive and entertaining as well.

> **Review Video: Descriptive Texts**
> Visit mometrix.com/academy and enter code: 174903

Expression of Feelings

When an author intends to **express feelings**, he or she may use **expressive and bold language**. An author may write with emotion for any number of reasons. Sometimes, authors will express feelings because they are describing a personal situation of great pain or happiness. In other situations, authors will attempt to persuade the reader and will use emotion to stir up the passions. This kind of expression is easy to identify when the writer uses phrases like *I felt* and *I sense*. However, readers may find that the author will simply describe feelings without introducing them. As a reader, you must know the importance of recognizing when an author is expressing emotion and not to become overwhelmed by sympathy or passion. Readers should maintain some

detachment so that they can still evaluate the strength of the author's argument or the quality of the writing.

Review Video: Emotional Language in Literature
Visit mometrix.com/academy and enter code: 759390

Expository Passage

An **expository** passage aims to **inform** and enlighten readers. Expository passages are nonfiction and usually center around a simple, easily defined topic. Since the goal of exposition is to teach, such a passage should be as clear as possible. Often, an expository passage contains helpful organizing words, like *first, next, for example*, and *therefore*. These words keep the reader **oriented** in the text. Although expository passages do not need to feature colorful language and artful writing, they are often more effective with these features. For a reader, the challenge of expository passages is to maintain steady attention. Expository passages are not always about subjects that will naturally interest a reader, so the writer is often more concerned with **clarity** and **comprehensibility** than with engaging the reader. By reading actively, you can ensure a good habit of focus when reading an expository passage.

Review Video: Expository Passages
Visit mometrix.com/academy and enter code: 256515

Narrative Passage

A **narrative** passage is a story that can be fiction or nonfiction. However, there are a few elements that a text must have in order to be classified as a narrative. First, the text must have a **plot** (i.e., a series of events). Narratives often proceed in a clear sequence, but this is not a requirement. If the narrative is good, then these events will be interesting to readers. Second, a narrative has **characters**. These characters could be people, animals, or even inanimate objects—so long as they participate in the plot. Third, a narrative passage often contains **figurative language** which is meant to stimulate the imagination of readers by making comparisons and observations. For instance, a *metaphor*, a common piece of figurative language, is a description of one thing in terms of another. *The moon was a frosty snowball* is an example of a metaphor. In the literal sense this is obviously untrue, but the comparison suggests a certain mood for the reader.

Technical Passage

A **technical** passage is written to *describe* a complex object or process. Technical writing is common in medical and technological fields, in which complex ideas of mathematics, science, and engineering need to be explained *simply* and *clearly*. To ease comprehension, a technical passage usually proceeds in a very logical order. Technical passages often have clear headings and subheadings, which are used to keep the reader oriented in the text. Additionally, you will find that these passages divide sections up with numbers or letters. Many technical passages look more like an outline than a piece of prose. The amount of **jargon** or difficult vocabulary will vary in a technical passage depending on the intended audience. As much as possible, technical passages try to avoid language that the reader will have to research in order to understand the message, yet readers will find that jargon cannot always be avoided.

Review Video: Technical Passages
Visit mometrix.com/academy and enter code: 478923

Common Organizations of Texts

ORGANIZATION OF THE TEXT

The way a text is organized can help readers understand the author's intent and his or her conclusions. There are various ways to organize a text, and each one has a purpose and use. Usually, authors will organize information logically in a passage so the reader can follow and locate the information within the text. However, since not all passages are written with the same logical structure, you need to be familiar with several different types of passage structure.

Review Video: Sequence of Events in a Story
Visit mometrix.com/academy and enter code: 807512

CHRONOLOGICAL

When using **chronological** order, the author presents information in the order that it happened. For example, biographies are typically written in chronological order. The subject's birth and childhood are presented first, followed by their adult life, and lastly the events leading up to the person's death.

CAUSE AND EFFECT

One of the most common text structures is **cause and effect**. A **cause** is an act or event that makes something happen, and an **effect** is the thing that happens as a result of the cause. A cause-and-effect relationship is not always explicit, but there are some terms in English that signal causes, such as *since*, *because*, and *due to*. Furthermore, terms that signal effects include *consequently, therefore, this leads to*. As an example, consider the sentence *Because the sky was clear, Ron did not bring an umbrella*. The cause is the clear sky, and the effect is that Ron did not bring an umbrella. However, readers may find that sometimes the cause-and-effect relationship will not be clearly noted. For instance, the sentence *He was late and missed the meeting* does not contain any signaling words, but the sentence still contains a cause (he was late) and an effect (he missed the meeting).

Review Video: Cause and Effect
Visit mometrix.com/academy and enter code: 868099

Review Video: Rhetorical Strategy of Cause and Effect Analysis
Visit mometrix.com/academy and enter code: 725944

MULTIPLE EFFECTS

Be aware of the possibility for a single cause to have **multiple effects.** (e.g., *Single cause*: Because you left your homework on the table, your dog engulfed the assignment. *Multiple effects*: As a result, you receive a failing grade, your parents do not allow you to go out with your friends, you miss out on the new movie, and one of your classmates spoils it for you before you have another chance to watch it).

MULTIPLE CAUSES

Also, there is the possibility for a single effect to have **multiple causes.** (e.g., *Single effect*: Alan has a fever. *Multiple causes*: An unexpected cold front came through the area, and Alan forgot to take his multi-vitamin to avoid getting sick.) Additionally, an effect can in turn be the cause of another effect, in what is known as a cause-and-effect chain. (e.g., As a result of her disdain for procrastination, Lynn prepared for her exam. This led to her passing her test with high marks. Hence, her resume was accepted and her application was approved.)

Cause and Effect in Persuasive Essays

Persuasive essays, in which an author tries to make a convincing argument and change the minds of readers, usually include cause-and-effect relationships. However, these relationships should not always be taken at face value. Frequently, an author will assume a cause or take an effect for granted. To read a persuasive essay effectively, readers need to judge the cause-and-effect relationships that the author is presenting. For instance, imagine an author wrote the following: *The parking deck has been unprofitable because people would prefer to ride their bikes.* The relationship is clear: the cause is that people prefer to ride their bikes, and the effect is that the parking deck has been unprofitable. However, readers should consider whether this argument is conclusive. Perhaps there are other reasons for the failure of the parking deck: a down economy, excessive fees, etc. Too often, authors present causal relationships as if they are fact rather than opinion. Readers should be on the alert for these dubious claims.

Problem-Solution

Some nonfiction texts are organized to **present a problem** followed by a solution. For this type of text, the problem is often explained before the solution is offered. In some cases, as when the problem is well known, the solution may be introduced briefly at the beginning. Other passages may focus on the solution, and the problem will be referenced only occasionally. Some texts will outline multiple solutions to a problem, leaving readers to choose among them. If the author has an interest or an allegiance to one solution, he or she may fail to mention or describe accurately some of the other solutions. Readers should be careful of the author's agenda when reading a problem-solution text. Only by understanding the author's perspective and interests can one develop a proper judgment of the proposed solution.

Compare and Contrast

Many texts follow the **compare-and-contrast** model in which the similarities and differences between two ideas or things are explored. Analysis of the similarities between ideas is called **comparison**. In an ideal comparison, the author places ideas or things in an equivalent structure, i.e., the author presents the ideas in the same way. If an author wants to show the similarities between cricket and baseball, then he or she may do so by summarizing the equipment and rules for each game. Be mindful of the similarities as they appear in the passage and take note of any differences that are mentioned. Often, these small differences will only reinforce the more general similarity.

Review Video: Compare and Contrast
Visit mometrix.com/academy and enter code: 798319

Thinking critically about ideas and conclusions can seem like a daunting task. One way to ease this task is to understand the basic elements of ideas and writing techniques. Looking at the ways different ideas relate to each other can be a good way for readers to begin their analysis. For instance, sometimes authors will write about two ideas that are in opposition to each other. Or, one author will provide his or her ideas on a topic, and another author may respond in opposition. The analysis of these opposing ideas is known as **contrast**. Contrast is often marred by the author's obvious partiality to one of the ideas. A discerning reader will be put off by an author who does not engage in a fair fight. In an analysis of opposing ideas, both ideas should be presented in clear and reasonable terms. If the author does prefer a side, you need to read carefully to determine the areas where the author shows or avoids this preference. In an analysis of opposing ideas, you should proceed through the passage by marking the major differences point by point with an eye that is looking for an explanation of each side's view. For instance, in an analysis of capitalism and communism, there is an importance in outlining each side's view on labor, markets, prices, personal responsibility, etc. Additionally, as you read through the passages, you should note whether the opposing views present each side in a similar manner.

SEQUENCE

Readers must be able to identify a text's **sequence**, or the order in which things happen. Often, when the sequence is very important to the author, the text is indicated with signal words like *first*, *then*, *next*, and *last*. However, a sequence can be merely implied and must be noted by the reader. Consider the sentence *He walked through the garden and gave water and fertilizer to the plants.* Clearly, the man did not walk through the garden before he collected water and fertilizer for the plants. So, the implied sequence is that he first collected water, then he collected fertilizer, next he walked through the garden, and last he gave water or fertilizer as necessary to the plants. Texts do not always proceed in an orderly sequence from first to last. Sometimes they begin at the end and start over at the beginning. As a reader, you can enhance your understanding of the passage by taking brief notes to clarify the sequence.

Review Video: Sequence
Visit mometrix.com/academy and enter code: 489027

Making and Evaluating Predictions

MAKING PREDICTIONS

When we read literature, **making predictions** about what will happen in the writing reinforces our purpose for reading and prepares us mentally. A **prediction** is a guess about what will happen next. Readers constantly make predictions based on what they have read and what they already know. We can make predictions before we begin reading and during our reading. Consider the following sentence: *Staring at the computer screen in shock, Kim blindly reached over for the brimming glass of water on the shelf to her side.* The sentence suggests that Kim is distracted, and that she is not looking at the glass that she is going to pick up. So, a reader might predict that Kim is going to knock over the glass. Of course, not every prediction will be accurate: perhaps Kim will pick the glass up cleanly. Nevertheless, the author has certainly created the expectation that the water might be spilled.

As we read on, we can test the accuracy of our predictions, revise them in light of additional reading, and confirm or refute our predictions. Predictions are always subject to revision as the reader acquires more information. A reader can make predictions by observing the title and illustrations; noting the structure, characters, and subject; drawing on existing knowledge relative to the subject; and asking "why" and "who" questions. Connecting reading to what we already know enables us to learn new information and construct meaning. For example, before third-graders read a book about Johnny Appleseed, they may start a KWL chart—a list of what they *Know*, what they *Want* to know or learn, and what they have *Learned* after reading. Activating existing background knowledge and thinking about the text before reading improves comprehension.

Review Video: Predictive Reading
Visit mometrix.com/academy and enter code: 437248

Test-taking tip: To respond to questions requiring future predictions, your answers should be based on evidence of past or present behavior and events.

Evaluating Predictions

When making predictions, readers should be able to explain how they developed their prediction. One way readers can defend their thought process is by citing textual evidence. Textual evidence to evaluate reader predictions about literature includes specific synopses of the work, paraphrases of the work or parts of it, and direct quotations from the work. These references to the text must support the prediction by indicating, clearly or unclearly, what will happen later in the story. A text may provide these indications through literary devices such as foreshadowing. Foreshadowing is anything in a text that gives the reader a hint about what is to come by emphasizing the likelihood of an event or development. Foreshadowing can occur through descriptions, exposition, and dialogue. Foreshadowing in dialogue usually occurs when a character gives a warning or expresses a strong feeling that a certain event will occur. Foreshadowing can also occur through irony. However, unlike other forms of foreshadowing, the events that seem the most likely are the opposite of what actually happens. Instances of foreshadowing and irony can be summarized, paraphrased, or quoted to defend a reader's prediction.

Review Video: Textual Evidence for Predictions
Visit mometrix.com/academy and enter code: 261070

Making Inferences and Drawing Conclusions

Inferences are logical conclusions that readers make based on their observations and previous knowledge. An inference is based on both what is found in a passage or a story and what is known from personal experience. For instance, a story may say that a character is frightened and can hear howling in the distance. Based on both what is in the text and personal knowledge, it is a logical conclusion that the character is frightened because he hears the sound of wolves. A good inference is supported by the information in a passage.

Implicit and Explicit Information

By inferring, readers construct meanings from text that are personally relevant. By combining their own schemas or concepts and their background information pertinent to the text with what they read, readers interpret it according to both what the author has conveyed and their own unique perspectives. Inferences are different from **explicit information**, which is clearly stated in a passage. Authors do not always explicitly spell out every meaning in what they write; many meanings are implicit. Through inference, readers can comprehend implied meanings in the text, and also derive personal significance from it, making the text meaningful and memorable to them. Inference is a natural process in everyday life. When readers infer, they can draw conclusions about what the author is saying, predict what may reasonably follow, amend these predictions as they continue to read, interpret the import of themes, and analyze the characters' feelings and motivations through their actions.

Example of Drawing Conclusions from Inferences

Read the excerpt and decide why Jana finally relaxed.

> Jana loved her job, but the work was very demanding. She had trouble relaxing. She called a friend, but she still thought about work. She ordered a pizza, but eating it did not help. Then, her kitten jumped on her lap and began to purr. Jana leaned back and began to hum a little tune. She felt better.

You can draw the conclusion that Jana relaxed because her kitten jumped on her lap. The kitten purred, and Jana leaned back and hummed a tune. Then she felt better. The excerpt does not explicitly say that this is the reason why she was able to relax. The text leaves the matter unclear, but the reader can infer or make a "best guess" that this is the reason she is relaxing. This is a logical conclusion based on the information in the passage. It is the best conclusion a reader can make based on the information he or she has read. Inferences are based on the information in a passage, but they are not directly stated in the passage.

Test-taking tip: While being tested on your ability to make correct inferences, you must look for **contextual clues**. An answer can be true, but not the best or most correct answer. The contextual clues will help you find the answer that is the **best answer** out of the given choices. Be careful in your reading to understand the context in which a phrase is stated. When asked for the implied meaning of a statement made in the passage, you should immediately locate the statement and read the **context** in which the statement was made. Also, look for an answer choice that has a similar phrase to the statement in question.

Review Video: Inference
Visit mometrix.com/academy and enter code: 379203

Review Video: How to Support a Conclusion
Visit mometrix.com/academy and enter code: 281653

Critical Reading Skills

Opinions, Facts, and Fallacies

Critical thinking skills are mastered through understanding various types of writing and the different purposes authors can have for writing different passages. Every author writes for a purpose. When you understand their purpose and how they accomplish their goal, you will be able to analyze their writing and determine whether or not you agree with their conclusions.

Readers must always be aware of the difference between fact and opinion. A **fact** can be subjected to analysis and proven to be true. An **opinion**, on the other hand, is the author's personal thoughts or feelings and may not be altered by research or evidence. If the author writes that the distance from New York City to Boston is about two hundred miles, then he or she is stating a fact. If the author writes that New York City is too crowded, then he or she is giving an opinion because there is no objective standard for overpopulation. Opinions are often supported by facts. For instance, an author might use a comparison between the population density of New York City and that of other major American cities as evidence of an overcrowded population. An opinion supported by facts tends to be more convincing. On the other hand, when authors support their opinions with other opinions, readers should employ critical thinking and approach the argument with skepticism.

Review Video: Distinguishing Fact and Opinion
Visit mometrix.com/academy and enter code: 870899

Reliable Sources

When you read an argumentative passage, you need to be sure that facts are presented to the reader from **reliable sources**. An opinion is what the author thinks about a given topic. An opinion is not common knowledge or proven by expert sources, instead the information is the personal beliefs and thoughts of the author. To distinguish between fact and opinion, a reader needs to consider the type of source that is presenting information, the information that backs-up a claim, and the author's motivation to have a certain point-of-view on a given topic. For example, if a panel of scientists has conducted multiple studies on the effectiveness of taking a certain vitamin, then the results are more likely to be factual than those of a company that is selling a vitamin and simply claims that taking the vitamin can produce positive effects. The company is motivated to sell their product, and the scientists are using the scientific method to prove a theory. Remember, if you find sentences that contain phrases such as "I think...", then the statement is an opinion.

Biases

In their attempts to persuade, writers often make mistakes in their thought processes and writing choices. These processes and choices are important to understand so you can make an informed decision about the author's credibility. Every author has a point of view, but authors demonstrate a **bias** when they ignore reasonable counterarguments or distort opposing viewpoints. A bias is evident whenever the author's claims are presented in a way that is unfair or inaccurate. Bias can be intentional or unintentional, but readers should be skeptical of the author's argument in either case. Remember that a biased author may still be correct. However, the author will be correct in spite of, not because of, his or her bias.

A **stereotype** is a bias applied specifically to a group of people or a place. Stereotyping is considered to be particularly abhorrent because it promotes negative, misleading generalizations about people. Readers should be very cautious of authors who use stereotypes in their writing. These faulty assumptions typically reveal the author's ignorance and lack of curiosity.

> **Review Video: Bias and Stereotype**
> Visit mometrix.com/academy and enter code: 644829

Reading Comprehension and Connecting with Texts

Comparing Two Stories

When presented with two different stories, there will be **similarities** and **differences** between the two. A reader needs to make a list, or other graphic organizer, of the points presented in each story. Once the reader has written down the main point and supporting points for each story, the two sets of ideas can be compared. The reader can then present each idea and show how it is the same or different in the other story. This is called **comparing and contrasting ideas**.

The reader can compare ideas by stating, for example: "In Story 1, the author believes that humankind will one day land on Mars, whereas in Story 2, the author believes that Mars is too far away for humans to ever step foot on." Note that the two viewpoints are different in each story that the reader is comparing. A reader may state that: "Both stories discussed the likelihood of humankind landing on Mars." This statement shows how the viewpoint presented in both stories is based on the same topic, rather than how each viewpoint is different. The reader will complete a comparison of two stories with a conclusion.

> **Review Video: How to Compare and Contrast**
> Visit mometrix.com/academy and enter code: 833765

Outlining a Passage

As an aid to drawing conclusions, **outlining** the information contained in the passage should be a familiar skill to readers. An effective outline will reveal the structure of the passage and will lead to solid conclusions. An effective outline will have a title that refers to the basic subject of the text, though the title does not need to restate the main idea. In most outlines, the main idea will be the first major section. Each major idea in the passage will be established as the head of a category. For instance, the most common outline format calls for the main ideas of the passage to be indicated with Roman numerals. In an effective outline of this kind, each of the main ideas will be represented by a Roman numeral and none of the Roman numerals will designate minor details or secondary ideas. Moreover, all supporting ideas and details should be placed in the appropriate place on the outline. An outline does not need to include every detail listed in the text, but it should feature all of those that are central to the argument or message. Each of these details should be listed under the corresponding main idea.

Review Video: Outlining as an Aid to Drawing Conclusions
Visit mometrix.com/academy and enter code: 584445

Using Graphic Organizers

Ideas from a text can also be organized using **graphic organizers**. A graphic organizer is a way to simplify information and take key points from the text. A graphic organizer such as a timeline may have an event listed for a corresponding date on the timeline, while an outline may have an event listed under a key point that occurs in the text. Each reader needs to create the type of graphic organizer that works the best for him or her in terms of being able to recall information from a story. Examples include a spider-map, which takes a main idea from the story and places it in a bubble with supporting points branching off the main idea. An outline is useful for diagramming the main and supporting points of the entire story, and a Venn diagram compares and contrasts characteristics of two or more ideas.

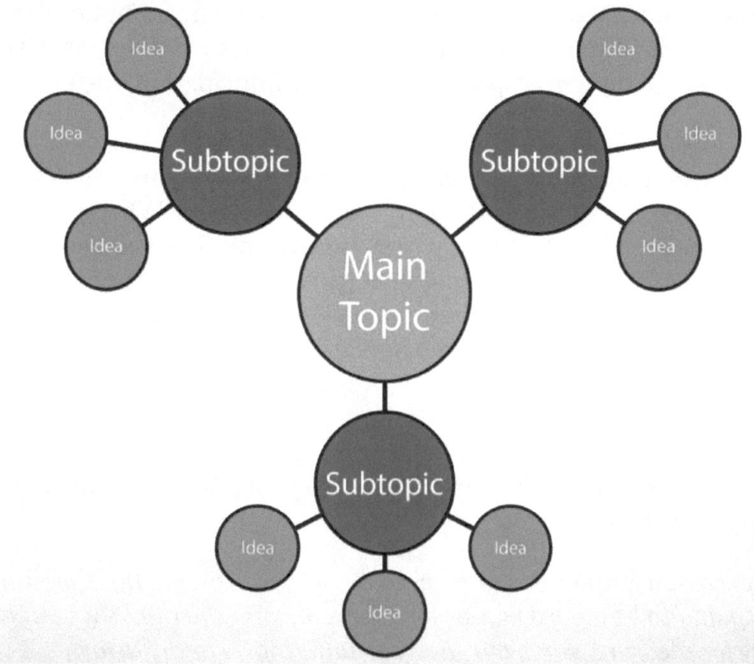

Review Video: Graphic Organizers
Visit mometrix.com/academy and enter code: 665513

Making Logical Conclusions about a Passage

A reader should always be drawing conclusions from the text. Sometimes conclusions are **implied** from written information, and other times the information is **stated directly** within the passage. One should always aim to draw conclusions from information stated within a passage, rather than to draw them from mere implications. At times an author may provide some information and then describe a counterargument. Readers should be alert for direct statements that are subsequently rejected or weakened by the author. Furthermore, you should always read through the entire passage before drawing conclusions. Many readers are trained to expect the author's conclusions at either the beginning or the end of the passage, but many texts do not adhere to this format.

Drawing conclusions from information implied within a passage requires confidence on the part of the reader. **Implications** are things that the author does not state directly, but readers can assume based on what the author does say. Consider the following passage: *I stepped outside and opened my umbrella. By the time I got to work, the cuffs of my pants were soaked.* The author never states that it is raining, but this fact is clearly implied. Conclusions based on implication must be well supported by the text. In order to draw a solid conclusion, readers should have **multiple pieces of evidence**. If readers have only one piece, they must be assured that there is no other possible explanation than their conclusion. A good reader will be able to draw many conclusions from information implied by the text, which will be a great help on the exam.

Drawing Conclusions

A common type of inference that a reader has to make is **drawing a conclusion**. The reader makes this conclusion based on the information provided within a text. Certain facts are included to help a reader come to a specific conclusion. For example, a story may open with a man trudging through the snow on a cold winter day, dragging a sled behind him. The reader can logically **infer** from the setting of the story that the man is wearing heavy winter clothes in order to stay warm. Information is implied based on the setting of a story, which is why **setting** is an important element of the text. If the same man in the example was trudging down a beach on a hot summer day, dragging a surf board behind him, the reader would assume that the man is not wearing heavy clothes. The reader makes inferences based on their own experiences and the information presented to them in the story.

Test-taking tip: When asked to identify a conclusion that may be drawn, look for critical "hedge" phrases, such as *likely*, *may*, *can*, and *will often*, among many others. When you are being tested on this knowledge, remember the question that writers insert into these hedge phrases to cover every possibility. Often an answer will be wrong simply because there is no room for exception. Extreme positive or negative answers (such as always or never) are usually not correct. When answering these questions, the reader **should not** use any outside knowledge that is not gathered directly or reasonably inferred from the passage. Correct answers can be derived straight from the passage.

Example

Read the following sentence from *Little Women* by Louisa May Alcott and draw a conclusion based upon the information presented:

> *You know the reason Mother proposed not having any presents this Christmas was because it is going to be a hard winter for everyone; and she thinks we ought not to spend money for pleasure, when our men are suffering so in the army.*

Based on the information in the sentence, the reader can conclude, or **infer**, that the men are away at war while the women are still at home. The pronoun *our* gives a clue to the reader that the character is speaking about men she knows. In addition, the reader can assume that the character is speaking to a brother or sister, since the term "Mother" is used by the character while speaking to another person. The reader can also come to the conclusion that the characters celebrate Christmas, since it is mentioned in the **context** of the sentence. In the sentence, the mother is presented as an unselfish character who is opinionated and thinks about the wellbeing of other people.

SUMMARIZING

A helpful tool is the ability to **summarize** the information that you have read in a paragraph or passage format. This process is similar to creating an effective outline. First, a summary should accurately define the main idea of the passage, though the summary does not need to explain this main idea in exhaustive detail. The summary should continue by laying out the most important supporting details or arguments from the passage. All of the significant supporting details should be included, and none of the details included should be irrelevant or insignificant. Also, the summary should accurately report all of these details. Too often, the desire for brevity in a summary leads to the sacrifice of clarity or accuracy. Summaries are often difficult to read because they omit all of the graceful language, digressions, and asides that distinguish great writing. However, an effective summary should communicate the same overall message as the original text.

Review Video: Summarizing Text
Visit mometrix.com/academy and enter code: 172903

PARAPHRASING

Paraphrasing is another method that the reader can use to aid in comprehension. When paraphrasing, one puts what they have read into their own words by rephrasing what the author has written, or one "translates" all of what the author shared into their own words by including as many details as they can.

EVALUATING A PASSAGE

It is important to understand the logical conclusion of the ideas presented in an informational text. **Identifying a logical conclusion** can help you determine whether you agree with the writer or not. Coming to this conclusion is much like making an inference: the approach requires you to combine the information given by the text with what you already know and make a logical conclusion. If the author intended for the reader to draw a certain conclusion, then you can expect the author's argumentation and detail to be leading in that direction.

One way to approach the task of drawing conclusions is to make brief **notes** of all the points made by the author. When the notes are arranged on paper, they may clarify the logical conclusion. Another way to approach conclusions is to consider whether the reasoning of the author raises any pertinent questions. Sometimes you will be able to draw several conclusions from a passage. On occasion these will be conclusions that were never imagined by the author. Therefore, be aware that these conclusions must be **supported directly by the text**.

EVALUATION OF SUMMARIES

A summary of a literary passage is a condensation in the reader's own words of the passage's main points. Several guidelines can be used in evaluating a summary. The summary should be complete yet concise. It should be accurate, balanced, fair, neutral, and objective, excluding the reader's own opinions or reactions. It should reflect in similar proportion how much each point summarized was covered in the original passage. Summary writers should include tags of attribution, like "Macaulay argues that" to reference the original author whose ideas are represented in the summary. Summary writers should not overuse quotations; they should only quote central concepts or phrases they cannot precisely convey in words other than those of the original author. Another aspect of evaluating a summary is considering whether it can stand alone as a coherent, unified composition. In addition, evaluation of a summary should include whether its writer has cited the original source of the passage they have summarized so that readers can find it.

Making Connections to Enhance Comprehension

Reading involves thinking. For good comprehension, readers make **text-to-self**, **text-to-text**, and **text-to-world connections**. Making connections helps readers understand text better and predict what might occur next based on what they already know, such as how characters in the story feel or what happened in another text. Text-to-self connections with the reader's life and experiences make literature more personally relevant and meaningful to readers. Readers can make connections before, during, and after reading—including whenever the text reminds them of something similar they have encountered in life or other texts. The genre, setting, characters, plot elements, literary structure and devices, and themes an author uses allow a reader to make connections to other works of literature or to people and events in their own lives. Venn diagrams and other graphic organizers help visualize connections. Readers can also make double-entry notes: key content, ideas, events, words, and quotations on one side, and the connections with these on the other.

Reading Argumentative Writing

Author's Argument in Argumentative Writing

In argumentative writing, the argument is a belief, position, or opinion that the author wants to convince readers to believe as well. For the first step, readers should identify the **issue**. Some issues are controversial, meaning people disagree about them. Gun control, foreign policy, and the death penalty are all controversial issues. The next step is to determine the **author's position** on the issue. That position or viewpoint constitutes the author's argument. Readers should then identify the **author's assumptions**: things he or she accepts, believes, or takes for granted without needing proof. Inaccurate or illogical assumptions produce flawed arguments and can mislead readers. Readers should identify what kinds of **supporting evidence** the author offers, such as research results, personal observations or experiences, case studies, facts, examples, expert testimony and opinions, and comparisons. Readers should decide how relevant this support is to the argument.

Review Video: Argumentative Writing
Visit mometrix.com/academy and enter code: 561544

Evaluating an Author's Argument

The first three reader steps to **evaluate an author's argument** are to identify the **author's assumptions**, identify the **supporting evidence**, and decide **whether the evidence is relevant**. For example, if an author is not an expert on a particular topic, then that author's personal experience or opinion might not be relevant. The fourth step is to assess the **author's objectivity**. For example, consider whether the author introduces clear, understandable supporting evidence and facts to support the argument. The fifth step is evaluating whether the author's **argument is complete**. When authors give sufficient support for their arguments and also anticipate and respond effectively to opposing arguments or objections to their points, their arguments are complete. However, some authors omit information that could detract from their arguments. If instead they stated this information and refuted it, it would strengthen their arguments. The sixth step in evaluating an author's argumentative writing is to assess whether the **argument is valid**. Providing clear, logical reasoning makes an author's argument valid. Readers should ask themselves whether the author's points follow a sequence that makes sense, and whether each point leads to the next. The seventh step is to determine whether the author's **argument is credible**, meaning that it is convincing and believable. Arguments that are not valid are not credible, so step seven depends on step six. Readers should be mindful of their own biases as they evaluate and should not expect authors to conclusively prove their arguments, but rather to provide effective support and reason.

Evaluating an Author's Method of Appeal

To evaluate the effectiveness of an appeal, it is important to consider the author's purpose for writing. Any appeals an author uses in their argument must be relevant to the argument's goal. For example, a writer that argues for the reclassification of Pluto, but primarily uses appeals to emotion, will not have an effective argument. This writer should focus on using appeals to logic and support their argument with provable facts. While most arguments should include appeals to logic, emotion, and credibility, some arguments only call for one or two of these types of appeal. Evidence can support an appeal, but the evidence must be relevant to truly strengthen the appeal's effectiveness. If the writer arguing for Pluto's reclassification uses the reasons for Jupiter's classification as evidence, their argument would be weak. This information may seem relevant because it is related to the classification of planets. However, this classification is highly dependent on the size of the celestial object, and Jupiter is significantly bigger than Pluto. This use of evidence is illogical and does not support the appeal. Even when appropriate evidence and appeals are used, appeals and arguments lose their effectiveness when they create logical fallacies.

Evidence

The term **text evidence** refers to information that supports a main point or minor points and can help lead the reader to a conclusion about the text's credibility. Information used as text evidence is precise, descriptive, and factual. A main point is often followed by supporting details that provide evidence to back up a claim. For example, a passage may include the claim that winter occurs during opposite months in the Northern and Southern hemispheres. Text evidence for this claim may include examples of countries where winter occurs in opposite months. Stating that the tilt of the Earth as it rotates around the sun causes winter to occur at different times in separate hemispheres is another example of text evidence. Text evidence can come from common knowledge, but it is also valuable to include text evidence from credible, relevant outside sources.

Review Video: Textual Evidence
Visit mometrix.com/academy and enter code: 486236

Evidence that supports the thesis and additional arguments needs to be provided. Most arguments must be supported by facts or statistics. A fact is something that is known with certainty, has been verified by several independent individuals, and can be proven to be true. In addition to facts, examples and illustrations can support an argument by adding an emotional component. With this component, you persuade readers in ways that facts and statistics cannot. The emotional component is effective when used alongside objective information that can be confirmed.

Credibility

The text used to support an argument can be the argument's downfall if the text is not credible. A text is **credible**, or believable, when its author is knowledgeable and objective, or unbiased. The author's motivations for writing the text play a critical role in determining the credibility of the text and must be evaluated when assessing that credibility. Reports written about the ozone layer by an environmental scientist and a hairdresser will have a different level of credibility.

Review Video: Author Credibility
Visit mometrix.com/academy and enter code: 827257

Appeal to Emotion

Sometimes, authors will appeal to the reader's emotion in an attempt to persuade or to distract the reader from the weakness of the argument. For instance, the author may try to inspire the pity of the reader by delivering a heart-rending story. An author also might use the bandwagon approach, in which he suggests that his opinion is correct because it is held by the majority. Some authors resort to name-calling, in which insults and harsh words are delivered to the opponent in an attempt to distract. In advertising, a common appeal is the celebrity testimonial, in which a famous person endorses a product. Of course, the fact that a famous person likes something should not really mean anything to the reader. These and other emotional appeals are usually evidence of poor reasoning and a weak argument.

Review Video: Emotional Language in Literature
Visit mometrix.com/academy and enter code: 759390

Counter Arguments

When authors give both sides to the argument, they build trust with their readers. As a reader, you should start with an undecided or neutral position. If an author presents only his or her side to the argument, then they are not exhibiting credibility and are weakening their argument.

Building common ground with readers can be effective for persuading neutral, skeptical, or opposed readers. Sharing values with undecided readers can allow people to switch positions without giving up what they feel is important. People who may oppose a position need to feel that they can change their minds without betraying who they are as a person. This appeal to having an open mind can be a powerful tool in arguing a position without antagonizing other views. Objections can be countered on a point-by-point basis or in a summary paragraph. Be mindful of how an author points out flaws in counter arguments. If they are unfair to the other side of the argument, then you should lose trust with the author.

Chapter Quiz

Ready to see how well you retained what you just read? Scan the QR code to go directly to the chapter quiz interface for this study guide. If you're using a computer, simply visit the bonus page at **mometrix.com/bonus948/kaplannursing** and click the Chapter Quizzes link.

Vocabulary, Spelling, and Grammar

Transform passive reading into active learning! After immersing yourself in this chapter, put your comprehension to the test by taking a quiz. The insights you gained will stay with you longer this way. Scan the QR code to go directly to the chapter quiz interface for this study guide. If you're using a computer, simply visit the bonus page at **mometrix.com/bonus948/kaplannursing** and click the Chapter Quizzes link.

Parts of Speech

Nouns

A noun is a person, place, thing, or idea. The two main types of nouns are **common** and **proper** nouns. Nouns can also be categorized as abstract (i.e., general) or concrete (i.e., specific).

Common Nouns

Common nouns are generic names for people, places, and things. Common nouns are not usually capitalized.

Examples of common nouns:

> *People*: boy, girl, worker, manager
>
> *Places*: school, bank, library, home
>
> *Things*: dog, cat, truck, car

Review Video: Nouns
Visit mometrix.com/academy and enter code: 344028

Proper Nouns

Proper nouns name specific people, places, or things. All proper nouns are capitalized.

Examples of proper nouns:

> *People*: Abraham Lincoln, George Washington, Martin Luther King, Jr.
>
> *Places*: Los Angeles, California; New York; Asia
>
> *Things*: Statue of Liberty, Earth, Lincoln Memorial

Note: Some nouns can be either common or proper depending on their use. For example, when referring to the planet that we live on, *Earth* is a proper noun and is capitalized. When referring to the dirt, rocks, or land on our planet, *earth* is a common noun and is not capitalized.

General and Specific Nouns

General nouns are the names of conditions or ideas. **Specific nouns** name people, places, and things that are understood by using your senses.

General nouns:

Condition: beauty, strength

Idea: truth, peace

Specific nouns:

People: baby, friend, father

Places: town, park, city hall

Things: rainbow, cough, apple, silk, gasoline

Collective Nouns

Collective nouns are the names for a group of people, places, or things that may act as a whole. The following are examples of collective nouns: *class, company, dozen, group, herd, team,* and *public.* Collective nouns usually require an article, which denotes the noun as being a single unit. For instance, a choir is a group of singers. Even though there are many singers in a choir, the word choir is grammatically treated as a single unit. If we refer to the members of the group, and not the group itself, it is no longer a collective noun.

Incorrect: The *choir are* going to compete nationally this year.

Correct: The *choir is* going to compete nationally this year.

Incorrect: The *members* of the choir *is* competing nationally this year.

Correct: The *members* of the choir *are* competing nationally this year.

Pronouns

Pronouns are words that are used to stand in for nouns. A pronoun may be classified as personal, intensive, relative, interrogative, demonstrative, indefinite, and reciprocal.

Personal: *Nominative* is the case for nouns and pronouns that are the subject of a sentence. *Objective* is the case for nouns and pronouns that are an object in a sentence. *Possessive* is the case for nouns and pronouns that show possession or ownership.

Singular

	Nominative	Objective	Possessive
First Person	I	me	my, mine
Second Person	you	you	your, yours
Third Person	he, she, it	him, her, it	his, her, hers, its

Plural

	Nominative	Objective	Possessive
First Person	we	us	our, ours
Second Person	you	you	your, yours
Third Person	they	them	their, theirs

Intensive: I myself, you yourself, he himself, she herself, the (thing) itself, we ourselves, you yourselves, they themselves

Relative: which, who, whom, whose

Interrogative: what, which, who, whom, whose

Demonstrative: this, that, these, those

Indefinite: all, any, each, everyone, either/neither, one, some, several

Reciprocal: each other, one another

Review Video: Nouns and Pronouns
Visit mometrix.com/academy and enter code: 312073

VERBS

A verb is a word or group of words that indicates action or being. In other words, the verb shows something's action or state of being or the action that has been done to something. If you want to write a sentence, then you need a verb. Without a verb, you have no sentence.

TRANSITIVE AND INTRANSITIVE VERBS

A **transitive verb** is a verb whose action indicates a receiver. **Intransitive verbs** do not indicate a receiver of an action. In other words, the action of the verb does not point to an object.

Transitive: He drives a car. | She feeds the dog.

Intransitive: He runs every day. | She voted in the last election.

A dictionary will tell you whether a verb is transitive or intransitive. Some verbs can be transitive or intransitive.

ACTION VERBS AND LINKING VERBS

Action verbs show what the subject is doing. In other words, an action verb shows action. Unlike most types of words, a single action verb, in the right context, can be an entire sentence. **Linking verbs** link the subject of a sentence to a noun or pronoun, or they link a subject with an adjective. You always need a verb if you want a complete sentence. However, linking verbs on their own cannot be a complete sentence.

Common linking verbs include *appear, be, become, feel, grow, look, seem, smell, sound,* and *taste.* However, any verb that shows a condition and connects to a noun, pronoun, or adjective that describes the subject of a sentence is a linking verb.

Action: He sings. | Run! | Go! | I talk with him every day. | She reads.

Linking:

Incorrect: I am.

Correct: I am John. | The roses smell lovely. | I feel tired.

Note: Some verbs are followed by words that look like prepositions, but they are a part of the verb and a part of the verb's meaning. These are known as phrasal verbs, and examples include *call off*, *look up*, and *drop off*.

Review Video: Action Verbs and Linking Verbs
Visit mometrix.com/academy and enter code: 743142

VOICE

Transitive verbs may be in active voice or passive voice. The difference between active voice and passive voice is whether the subject is acting or being acted upon. When the subject of the sentence is doing the action, the verb is in **active voice**. When the subject is being acted upon, the verb is in **passive voice**.

Active: Jon drew the picture. (The subject *Jon* is doing the action of *drawing a picture*.)

Passive: The picture is drawn by Jon. (The subject *picture* is receiving the action from Jon.)

VERB TENSES

Verb **tense** is a property of a verb that indicates when the action being described takes place (past, present, or future) and whether or not the action is completed (simple or perfect). Describing an action taking place in the present (*I talk*) requires a different verb tense than describing an action that took place in the past (*I talked*). Some verb tenses require an auxiliary (helping) verb. These helping verbs include *am, are, is* | *have, has, had* | *was, were, will* (or *shall*).

Present: I talk	Present perfect: I have talked
Past: I talked	Past perfect: I had talked
Future: I will talk	Future perfect: I will have talked

Present: The action is happening at the current time.

Example: He *walks* to the store every morning.

To show that something is happening right now, use the progressive present tense: I *am walking*.

Past: The action happened in the past.

Example: She *walked* to the store an hour ago.

Future: The action will happen later.

Example: I *will walk* to the store tomorrow.

Present perfect: The action started in the past and continues into the present or took place previously at an unspecified time.

Example: I *have walked* to the store three times today.

Past perfect: The action was completed at some point in the past. This tense is usually used to describe an action that was completed before some other reference time or event.

Example: I *had eaten* already before they arrived.

Future perfect: The action will be completed before some point in the future. This tense may be used to describe an action that has already begun or has yet to begin.

Example: The project *will have been completed* by the deadline.

Review Video: Present Perfect, Past Perfect, and Future Perfect Verb Tenses
Visit mometrix.com/academy and enter code: 269472

Conjugating Verbs

When you need to change the form of a verb, you are **conjugating** a verb. The key forms of a verb are present tense (sing/sings), past tense (sang), present participle (singing), and past participle (sung). By combining these forms with helping verbs, you can make almost any verb tense. The following table demonstrate some of the different ways to conjugate a verb:

Tense	First Person	Second Person	Third Person Singular	Third Person Plural
Simple Present	I sing	You sing	He, she, it sings	They sing
Simple Past	I sang	You sang	He, she, it sang	They sang
Simple Future	I will sing	You will sing	He, she, it will sing	They will sing
Present Progressive	I am singing	You are singing	He, she, it is singing	They are singing
Past Progressive	I was singing	You were singing	He, she, it was singing	They were singing
Present Perfect	I have sung	You have sung	He, she, it has sung	They have sung
Past Perfect	I had sung	You had sung	He, she, it had sung	They had sung

Mood

There are three **moods** in English: the indicative, the imperative, and the subjunctive.

The **indicative mood** is used for facts, opinions, and questions.

Fact: You can do this.

Opinion: I think that you can do this.

Question: Do you know that you can do this?

The **imperative** is used for orders or requests.

Order: You are going to do this!

Request: Will you do this for me?

The **subjunctive mood** is for wishes and statements that go against fact.

Wish: I wish that I were famous.

Statement against fact: If I were you, I would do this. (This goes against fact because I am not you. You have the chance to do this, and I do not have the chance.)

ADJECTIVES

An **adjective** is a word that is used to modify a noun or pronoun. An adjective answers a question: *Which one? What kind?* or *How many?* Usually, adjectives come before the words that they modify, but they may also come after a linking verb.

Which one? The *third* suit is my favorite.

What kind? This suit is *navy blue.*

How many? I am going to buy *four* pairs of socks to match the suit.

> **Review Video: Descriptive Text**
> Visit mometrix.com/academy and enter code: 174903

ARTICLES

Articles are adjectives that are used to distinguish nouns as definite or indefinite. *A*, *an*, and *the* are the only articles. **Definite** nouns are preceded by *the* and indicate a specific person, place, thing, or idea. **Indefinite** nouns are preceded by *a* or *an* and do not indicate a specific person, place, thing, or idea.

Note: *An* comes before words that start with a vowel sound. For example, "Are you going to get an **u**mbrella?"

Definite: I lost *the* bottle that belongs to me.

Indefinite: Does anyone have *a* bottle to share?

> **Review Video: Function of Articles in a Sentence**
> Visit mometrix.com/academy and enter code: 449383

COMPARISON WITH ADJECTIVES

Some adjectives are relative and other adjectives are absolute. Adjectives that are **relative** can show the comparison between things. **Absolute** adjectives can also show comparison, but they do so in a different way. Let's say that you are reading two books. You think that one book is perfect, and the other book is not exactly perfect. It is not possible for one book to be more perfect than the other. Either you think that the book is perfect, or you think that the book is imperfect. In this case, perfect and imperfect are absolute adjectives.

Relative adjectives will show the different **degrees** of something or someone to something else or someone else. The three degrees of adjectives include positive, comparative, and superlative.

The **positive** degree is the normal form of an adjective.

Example: This work is *difficult.* | She is *smart.*

The **comparative** degree compares one person or thing to another person or thing.

Example: This work is *more difficult* than your work. | She is *smarter* than me.

The **superlative** degree compares more than two people or things.

Example: This is the *most difficult* work of my life. | She is the *smartest* lady in school.

Review Video: Adjectives
Visit mometrix.com/academy and enter code: 470154

ADVERBS

An **adverb** is a word that is used to **modify** a verb, an adjective, or another adverb. Usually, adverbs answer one of these questions: *When? Where? How?* and *Why?* The negatives *not* and *never* are considered adverbs. Adverbs that modify adjectives or other adverbs **strengthen** or **weaken** the words that they modify.

Examples:

He walks *quickly* through the crowd.

The water flows *smoothly* on the rocks.

Note: Adverbs are usually indicated by the morpheme *-ly*, which has been added to the root word. For instance, *quick* can be made into an adverb by adding *-ly* to construct *quickly*. Some words that end in *-ly* do not follow this rule and can behave as other parts of speech. Examples of adjectives ending in *-ly* include: *early, friendly, holy, lonely, silly*, and *ugly*. To know if a word that ends in *-ly* is an adjective or adverb, check your dictionary. Also, while many adverbs end in *-ly*, you need to remember that not all adverbs end in *-ly*.

Examples:

He is *never* angry.

You are *too* irresponsible to travel alone.

Review Video: Adverbs
Visit mometrix.com/academy and enter code: 713951

Review Video: Adverbs that Modify Adjectives
Visit mometrix.com/academy and enter code: 122570

COMPARISON WITH ADVERBS

The rules for comparing adverbs are the same as the rules for adjectives.

The **positive** degree is the standard form of an adverb.

Example: He arrives *soon*. | She speaks *softly* to her friends.

The **comparative** degree compares one person or thing to another person or thing.

Example: He arrives *sooner* than Sarah. | She speaks *more softly* than him.

The **superlative** degree compares more than two people or things.

Example: He arrives *soonest* of the group. | She speaks the *most softly* of any of her friends.

Prepositions

A **preposition** is a word placed before a noun or pronoun that shows the relationship between that noun or pronoun and another word in the sentence.

Common prepositions:

about	before	during	on	under
after	beneath	for	over	until
against	between	from	past	up
among	beyond	in	through	with
around	by	of	to	within
at	down	off	toward	without

Examples:

The napkin is *in* the drawer.

The Earth rotates *around* the Sun.

The needle is *beneath* the haystack.

Can you find "me" *among* the words?

Review Video: Prepositions
Visit mometrix.com/academy and enter code: 946763

Conjunctions

Conjunctions join words, phrases, or clauses and they show the connection between the joined pieces. **Coordinating conjunctions** connect equal parts of sentences. **Correlative conjunctions** show the connection between pairs. **Subordinating conjunctions** join subordinate (i.e., dependent) clauses with independent clauses.

Coordinating Conjunctions

The **coordinating conjunctions** include: *and, but, yet, or, nor, for,* and *so*

Examples:

The rock was small, *but* it was heavy.

She drove in the night, *and* he drove in the day.

Correlative Conjunctions

The **correlative conjunctions** are: *either...or* | *neither...nor* | *not only...but also*

Examples:

> *Either* you are coming *or* you are staying.
>
> He *not only* ran three miles *but also* swam 200 yards.

Review Video: Coordinating and Correlative Conjunctions
Visit mometrix.com/academy and enter code: 390329

Review Video: Adverb Equal Comparisons
Visit mometrix.com/academy and enter code: 231291

Subordinating Conjunctions

Common **subordinating conjunctions** include:

after	since	whenever
although	so that	where
because	unless	wherever
before	until	whether
in order that	when	while

Examples:

> I am hungry *because* I did not eat breakfast.
>
> He went home *when* everyone left.

Review Video: Subordinating Conjunctions
Visit mometrix.com/academy and enter code: 958913

Interjections

Interjections are words of exclamation (i.e., audible expression of great feeling) that are used alone or as a part of a sentence. Often, they are used at the beginning of a sentence for an introduction. Sometimes, they can be used in the middle of a sentence to show a change in thought or attitude.

> Common Interjections: Hey! | Oh, | Ouch! | Please! | Wow!

Agreement and Sentence Structure

Subjects and Predicates

Subjects

The **subject** of a sentence names who or what the sentence is about. The subject may be directly stated in a sentence, or the subject may be the implied *you*. The **complete subject** includes the simple subject and all of its modifiers. To find the complete subject, ask *Who* or *What* and insert the verb to complete the question. The answer, including any modifiers (adjectives, prepositional phrases, etc.), is the complete subject. To find the **simple subject**, remove all of the modifiers in the complete subject. Being able to locate the subject of a sentence helps with many problems, such as those involving sentence fragments and subject-verb agreement.

Examples:

The small, red car is the one that he wants for Christmas. (simple subject: car; complete subject: The small, red car)

The young artist is coming over for dinner. (simple subject: artist; complete subject: The young artist)

Review Video: Subjects in English
Visit mometrix.com/academy and enter code: 444771

In **imperative** sentences, the verb's subject is understood (e.g., [You] Run to the store), but is not actually present in the sentence. Normally, the subject comes before the verb. However, the subject comes after the verb in sentences that begin with *There are* or *There was*.

Direct:

John knows the way to the park.	Who knows the way to the park?	John
The cookies need ten more minutes.	What needs ten minutes?	The cookies
By five o'clock, Bill will need to leave.	Who needs to leave?	Bill
There are five letters on the table for him.	What is on the table?	Five letters
There were coffee and doughnuts in the house.	What was in the house?	Coffee and doughnuts

Implied:

Go to the post office for me.	Who is going to the post office?	You
Come and sit with me, please?	Who needs to come and sit?	You

PREDICATES

In a sentence, you always have a predicate and a subject. The subject tells who or what the sentence is about, and the **predicate** explains or describes the subject. The predicate includes the verb or verb phrase and any direct or indirect objects of the verb, as well as any words or phrases modifying these.

Think about the sentence *He sings*. In this sentence, we have a subject (He) and a predicate (sings). This is all that is needed for a sentence to be complete. Most sentences contain more information, but if this is all the information that you are given, then you have a complete sentence.

Now, let's look at another sentence: *John and Jane sing on Tuesday nights at the dance hall.*

subject: John and Jane | predicate: sing on Tuesday nights at the dance hall.

John and Jane sing on Tuesday nights at the dance hall.

Review Video: Complete Predicate
Visit mometrix.com/academy and enter code: 293942

SUBJECT-VERB AGREEMENT

Verbs must **agree** with their subjects in number and in person. To agree in number, singular subjects need singular verbs and plural subjects need plural verbs. A **singular** noun refers to **one** person, place, or thing. A **plural** noun refers to **more than one** person, place, or thing. To agree in person, the correct verb form must be chosen to match the first, second, or third person subject. The present tense ending *-s* or *-es* is used on a verb if its subject is third person singular; otherwise, the verb's ending is not modified.

Review Video: Subject-Verb Agreement
Visit mometrix.com/academy and enter code: 479190

NUMBER AGREEMENT EXAMPLES:

singular subject: Dan | singular verb: calls

Single Subject and Verb: Dan calls home.

Dan is one person. So, the singular verb *calls* is needed.

plural subject: Dan and Bob | plural verb: call

Plural Subject and Verb: Dan and Bob call home.

More than one person needs the plural verb *call*.

PERSON AGREEMENT EXAMPLES:

First Person: I *am* walking.

Second Person: You *are* walking.

Third Person: He *is* walking.

COMPLICATIONS WITH SUBJECT-VERB AGREEMENT

WORDS BETWEEN SUBJECT AND VERB

Words that come between the simple subject and the verb have no bearing on subject-verb agreement.

Examples:

singular subject: joy | singular verb: returns

The joy of my life returns home tonight.

The phrase *of my life* does not influence the verb *returns.*

singular subject: question; singular verb: is

The question that still remains unanswered is "Who are you?"

Don't let the phrase "*that still remains...*" trouble you. The subject *question* goes with *is.*

Compound Subjects

A compound subject is formed when two or more nouns joined by *and, or,* or *nor* jointly act as the subject of the sentence.

Joined by And

When a compound subject is joined by *and,* it is treated as a plural subject and requires a plural verb.

Examples:

plural subject: You and Jon; plural verb: are

You and Jon are invited to come to my house.

plural subject: pencil and paper; plural verb: belong

The pencil and paper belong to me.

Joined by Or/Nor

For a compound subject joined by *or* or *nor,* the verb must agree in number with the part of the subject that is closest to the verb (italicized in the examples below).

Examples:

subject: Today or tomorrow; verb: is

Today or tomorrow is the day.

subject: Stan or Phil; verb: wants

Stan or Phil wants to read the book.

subject: the pen nor the book; verb: is

Neither the pen nor the book is on the desk.

subject: blanket or pillows; verb: arrive

Either the blanket or pillows arrive this afternoon.

Indefinite Pronouns as Subject

An indefinite pronoun is a pronoun that does not refer to a specific noun. Some indefinite pronouns function as only singular, some function as only plural, and some can function as either singular or plural depending on how they are used.

Always Singular

Pronouns such as *each*, *either*, *everybody*, *anybody*, *somebody*, and *nobody* are always singular.

Examples:

Each (singular subject) of the runners has (singular verb) a different bib number.

Is (singular verb) either (singular subject) of you ready for the game?

Note: The words *each* and *either* can also be used as adjectives (e.g., *each* person is unique). When one of these adjectives modifies the subject of a sentence, it is always a singular subject.

Everybody (singular subject) grows (singular verb) a day older every day.

Anybody (singular subject) is (singular verb) welcome to bring a tent.

Always Plural

Pronouns such as *both*, *several*, and *many* are always plural.

Examples:

Both (plural subject) of the siblings were (plural verb) too tired to argue.

Many (plural subject) have tried (plural verb), but none have succeeded.

Depend on Context

Pronouns such as *some*, *any*, *all*, *none*, *more*, and *most* can be either singular or plural depending on what they are representing in the context of the sentence.

Examples:

All (singular subject) of my dog's food was (singular verb) still there in his bowl.

By the end of the night, all (plural subject) of my guests were (plural verb) already excited about coming to my next party.

Other Cases Involving Plural or Irregular Form

Some nouns are **singular in meaning but plural in form**: news, mathematics, physics, and economics.

The *news is* coming on now.

Mathematics is my favorite class.

Some nouns are plural in form and meaning, and have **no singular equivalent**: scissors and pants.

Do these *pants come* with a shirt?

The *scissors are* for my project.

Mathematical operations are **irregular** in their construction, but are normally considered to be **singular in meaning**.

One plus one is two.

Three times three is nine.

Note: Look to your **dictionary** for help when you aren't sure whether a noun with a plural form has a singular or plural meaning.

Complements

A complement is a noun, pronoun, or adjective that is used to give more information about the subject or object in the sentence.

Direct Objects

A direct object is a noun or pronoun that tells who or what **receives** the action of the verb. A sentence will only include a direct object if the verb is a transitive verb. If the verb is an intransitive verb or a linking verb, there will be no direct object. When you are looking for a direct object, find the verb and ask *who* or *what.*

Examples:

I took *the blanket.*

Jane read *books.*

Indirect Objects

An indirect object is a noun or pronoun that indicates what or whom the action had an **influence** on. If there is an indirect object in a sentence, then there will also be a direct object. When you are looking for the indirect object, find the verb and ask *to/for whom or what*.

Examples:

We taught [the old dog]indirect object [a new trick]direct object.

I gave [them]indirect object [a math lesson]direct object.

Review Video: Direct and Indirect Objects
Visit mometrix.com/academy and enter code: 817385

Predicate Nominatives and Predicate Adjectives

As we looked at previously, verbs may be classified as either action verbs or linking verbs. A linking verb is so named because it links the subject to words in the predicate that describe or define the subject. These words are called predicate nominatives (if nouns or pronouns) or predicate adjectives (if adjectives).

Examples:

My [father]subject is a [lawyer]predicate nominative.

Your [mother]subject is [patient]predicate adjective.

Pronoun Usage

The **antecedent** is the noun that has been replaced by a pronoun. A pronoun and its antecedent **agree** when they have the same number (singular or plural) and gender (male, female, or neutral).

Examples:

Singular agreement: [John]antecedent came into town, and [he]pronoun played for us.

Plural agreement: [John and Rick]antecedent came into town, and [they]pronoun played for us.

To determine which is the correct pronoun to use in a compound subject or object, try each pronoun **alone** in place of the compound in the sentence. Your knowledge of pronouns will tell you which one is correct.

Vocabulary, Spelling, and Grammar

Example:

Bob and (I, me) will be going.

Test: (1) *I will be going* or (2) *Me will be going*. The second choice cannot be correct because *me* cannot be used as the subject of a sentence. Instead, *me* is used as an object.

Answer: Bob and I will be going.

When a pronoun is used with a noun immediately following (as in "we boys"), try the sentence **without the added noun**.

Example:

(We/Us) boys played football last year.

Test: (1) *We played football last ye*ar or (2) *Us played football last year*. Again, the second choice cannot be correct because *us* cannot be used as a subject of a sentence. Instead, *us* is used as an object.

Answer: We boys played football last year.

Review Video: Pronoun Usage
Visit mometrix.com/academy and enter code: 666500

Review Video: Pronoun-Antecedent Agreement
Visit mometrix.com/academy and enter code: 919704

A pronoun should point clearly to the **antecedent**. Here is how a pronoun reference can be unhelpful if it is puzzling or not directly stated.

Unhelpful: Ron and Jim (antecedent) went to the store, and he (pronoun) bought soda.

Who bought soda? Ron or Jim?

Helpful: Jim (antecedent) went to the store, and he (pronoun) bought soda.

The sentence is clear. Jim bought the soda.

Some pronouns change their form by their placement in a sentence. A pronoun that is a **subject** in a sentence comes in the **subjective case**. Pronouns that serve as **objects** appear in the **objective case**. Finally, the pronouns that are used as **possessives** appear in the **possessive case**.

Examples:

Subjective case: *He* is coming to the show.

The pronoun *He* is the subject of the sentence.

Objective case: Josh drove *him* to the airport.

The pronoun *him* is the object of the sentence.

Possessive case: The flowers are *mine*.

The pronoun *mine* shows ownership of the flowers.

The word *who* is a subjective-case pronoun that can be used as a **subject**. The word *whom* is an objective-case pronoun that can be used as an **object**. The words *who* and *whom* are common in subordinate clauses or in questions.

Examples:

He knows who (subject) wants (verb) to come.

He knows the man whom (object) we want (verb) at the party.

Clauses

A clause is a group of words that contains both a subject and a predicate (verb). There are two types of clauses: independent and dependent. An **independent clause** contains a complete thought, while a **dependent (or subordinate) clause** does not. A dependent clause includes a subject and a verb, and may also contain objects or complements, but it cannot stand as a complete thought without being joined to an independent clause. Dependent clauses function within sentences as adjectives, adverbs, or nouns.

Example:

I am running (independent clause) because I want to stay in shape. (dependent clause)

The clause *I am running* is an independent clause: it has a subject and a verb, and it gives a complete thought. The clause *because I want to stay in shape* is a dependent clause: it has a subject and a verb, but it does not express a complete thought. It adds detail to the independent clause to which it is attached.

Review Video: Clauses
Visit mometrix.com/academy and enter code: 940170

Review Video: Independent and Dependent Clauses
Visit mometrix.com/academy and enter code: 556903

Types of Dependent Clauses

Adjective Clauses

An **adjective clause** is a dependent clause that modifies a noun or a pronoun. Adjective clauses begin with a relative pronoun (*who, whose, whom, which,* and *that*) or a relative adverb (*where, when,* and *why*).

Also, adjective clauses usually come immediately after the noun that the clause needs to explain or rename. This is done to ensure that it is clear which noun or pronoun the clause is modifying.

Examples:

independent clause: I learned the reason | adjective clause: why I won the award.

independent clause: This is the place | adjective clause: where I started my first job.

An adjective clause can be an essential or nonessential clause. An essential clause is very important to the sentence. **Essential clauses** explain or define a person or thing. **Nonessential clauses** give more information about a person or thing but are not necessary to define them. Nonessential clauses are set off with commas while essential clauses are not.

Examples:

A person [essential clause: who works hard at first] can often rest later in life.

Neil Armstrong, [nonessential clause: who walked on the moon,] is my hero.

Review Video: Adjective Clauses and Phrases
Visit mometrix.com/academy and enter code: 520888

Adverb Clauses

An **adverb clause** is a dependent clause that modifies a verb, adjective, or adverb. In sentences with multiple dependent clauses, adverb clauses are usually placed immediately before or after the independent clause. An adverb clause is introduced with words such as *after, although, as, before, because, if, since, so, unless, when, where*, and *while*.

Examples:

[adverb clause: When you walked outside,] I called the manager.

I will go with you [adverb clause: unless you want to stay.]

Noun Clauses

A **noun clause** is a dependent clause that can be used as a subject, object, or complement. Noun clauses begin with words such as *how, that, what, whether, which, who,* and *why*. These words can also come with an adjective clause. Unless the noun clause is being used as the subject of the sentence, it should come after the verb of the independent clause.

Examples:

noun clause

The real mystery is how you avoided serious injury.

noun clause

What you learn from each other depends on your honesty with others.

Subordination

When two related ideas are not of equal importance, the ideal way to combine them is to make the more important idea an independent clause and the less important idea a dependent or subordinate clause. This is called **subordination**.

Example:

> **Separate ideas**: The team had a perfect regular season. The team lost the championship.
>
> **Subordinated**: Despite having a perfect regular season, *the team lost the championship.*

Phrases

A phrase is a group of words that functions as a single part of speech, usually a noun, adjective, or adverb. A **phrase** is not a complete thought and does not contain a subject and predicate, but it adds detail or explanation to a sentence, or renames something within the sentence.

Prepositional Phrases

One of the most common types of phrases is the prepositional phrase. A **prepositional phrase** begins with a preposition and ends with a noun or pronoun that is the object of the preposition. Normally, the prepositional phrase functions as an **adjective** or an **adverb** within the sentence.

Examples:

prepositional phrase

The picnic is on the blanket.

prepositional phrase

I am sick with a fever today.

prepositional phrase

Among the many flowers, John found a four-leaf clover.

Verbal Phrases

A **verbal** is a word or phrase that is formed from a verb but does not function as a verb. Depending on its particular form, it may be used as a noun, adjective, or adverb. A verbal does **not** replace a verb in a sentence.

Examples:

verb

Correct: Walk a mile daily.

This is a complete sentence with the implied subject *you*.

Incorrect: To walk (verbal) a mile.

This is not a sentence since there is no functional verb.

There are three types of verbal: **participles**, **gerunds**, and **infinitives**. Each type of verbal has a corresponding **phrase** that consists of the verbal itself along with any complements or modifiers.

PARTICIPLES

A **participle** is a type of verbal that always functions as an adjective. The present participle always ends with *-ing*. Past participles end with *-d, -ed, -n,* or *-t*. Participles are combined with helping verbs to form certain verb tenses, but a participle by itself cannot function as a verb.

Examples: dance (verb) | dancing (present participle) | danced (past participle)

Participial phrases most often come right before or right after the noun or pronoun that they modify.

Examples:

Shipwrecked on an island, (participial phrase) the boys started to fish for food.

Having been seated for five hours, (participial phrase) we got out of the car to stretch our legs.

Praised for their work, (participial phrase) the group accepted the first-place trophy.

GERUNDS

A **gerund** is a type of verbal that always functions as a **noun**. Like present participles, gerunds always end with *-ing*, but they can be easily distinguished from participles by the part of speech they represent (participles always function as adjectives). Since a gerund or gerund phrase always functions as a noun, it can be used as the subject of a sentence, the predicate nominative, or the object of a verb or preposition.

Examples:

We want to be known for teaching (gerund) the poor (object of preposition: teaching the poor).

Coaching (gerund) this team (subject: Coaching this team) is the best job of my life.

We like practicing (gerund) our songs (object of verb: practicing our songs) in the basement.

Infinitives

An **infinitive** is a type of verbal that can function as a noun, an adjective, or an adverb. An infinitive is made of the word *to* and the basic form of the verb. As with all other types of verbal phrases, an infinitive phrase includes the verbal itself and all of its complements or modifiers.

Examples:

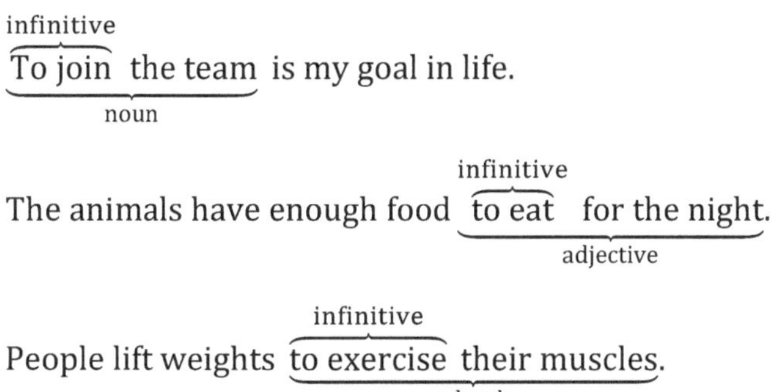

Review Video: Verbals
Visit mometrix.com/academy and enter code: 915480

Appositive Phrases

An **appositive** is a word or phrase that is used to explain or rename nouns or pronouns. Noun phrases, gerund phrases, and infinitive phrases can all be used as appositives.

Examples:

appositive
Terriers, hunters at heart, have been dressed up to look like lap dogs.

The noun phrase *hunters at heart* renames the noun *terriers.*

appositive
His plan, to save and invest his money, was proven as a safe approach.

The infinitive phrase explains what the plan is.

Appositive phrases can be **essential** or **nonessential**. An appositive phrase is essential if the person, place, or thing being described or renamed is too general for its meaning to be understood without the appositive.

Examples:

essential
Two of America's Founding Fathers, George Washington and Thomas Jefferson, served as presidents.

nonessential
George Washington and Thomas Jefferson, two Founding Fathers, served as presidents.

Absolute Phrases

An absolute phrase is a phrase that consists of **a noun followed by a participle**. An absolute phrase provides **context** to what is being described in the sentence, but it does not modify or explain any particular word; it is essentially independent.

Examples:

noun participle
The alarm ringing, he pushed the snooze button.
absolute phrase

noun participle
The music paused, she continued to dance through the crowd.
absolute phrase

Parallelism

When multiple items or ideas are presented in a sentence in series, such as in a list, the items or ideas must be stated in grammatically equivalent ways. For example, if two ideas are listed in parallel and the first is stated in gerund form, the second cannot be stated in infinitive form. (e.g., *I enjoy reading and to study.* [incorrect]) An infinitive and a gerund are not grammatically equivalent. Instead, you should write *I enjoy reading and studying* OR *I like to read and to study*. In lists of more than two, all items must be parallel.

Example:

> **Incorrect**: He stopped at the office, grocery store, and the pharmacy before heading home.
>
> The first and third items in the list of places include the article *the*, so the second item needs it as well.
>
> **Correct**: He stopped at the office, *the* grocery store, and the pharmacy before heading home.

Example:

> **Incorrect**: While vacationing in Europe, she went biking, skiing, and climbed mountains.
>
> The first and second items in the list are gerunds, so the third item must be as well.
>
> **Correct**: While vacationing in Europe, she went biking, skiing, and *mountain climbing.*

Review Video: Parallel Sentence Construction
Visit mometrix.com/academy and enter code: 831988

Sentence Purpose

There are four types of sentences: declarative, imperative, interrogative, and exclamatory.

A **declarative** sentence states a fact and ends with a period.

> *The football game starts at seven o'clock.*

An **imperative** sentence tells someone to do something and generally ends with a period. An urgent command might end with an exclamation point instead.

> *Don't forget to buy your ticket.*

An **interrogative** sentence asks a question and ends with a question mark.

> *Are you going to the game on Friday?*

An **exclamatory** sentence shows strong emotion and ends with an exclamation point.

> *I can't believe we won the game!*

SENTENCE STRUCTURE

Sentences are classified by structure based on the type and number of clauses present. The four classifications of sentence structure are the following:

Simple: A simple sentence has one independent clause with no dependent clauses. A simple sentence may have **compound elements** (i.e., compound subject or verb).

Examples:

single subject: Judy; single verb: watered

Judy watered the lawn.

compound subject: Judy and Alan; single verb: watered

Judy and Alan watered the lawn.

single subject: Judy; compound verb: watered … pulled

Judy watered the lawn and pulled weeds.

compound subject: Judy and Alan; compound verb: watered … pulled

Judy and Alan watered the lawn and pulled weeds.

Compound: A compound sentence has two or more independent clauses with no dependent clauses. Usually, the independent clauses are joined with a comma and a coordinating conjunction or with a semicolon.

Examples:

independent clause: The time has come,; independent clause: we are ready.

The time has come, and we are ready.

independent clause: I woke up at dawn;; independent clause: the sun was just coming up.

I woke up at dawn; the sun was just coming up.

Complex: A complex sentence has one independent clause and at least one dependent clause.

Examples:

Although he had the flu, (dependent clause) Harry went to work. (independent clause)

Marcia got married, (independent clause) after she finished college. (dependent clause)

Compound-Complex: A compound-complex sentence has at least two independent clauses and at least one dependent clause.

Examples:

John is my friend (independent clause) who went to India, (dependent clause) and he brought back souvenirs. (independent clause)

You may not realize this, (independent clause) but we heard the music (independent clause) that you played last night. (dependent clause)

Review Video: Sentence Structure
Visit mometrix.com/academy and enter code: 700478

Sentence variety is important to consider when writing an essay or speech. A variety of sentence lengths and types creates rhythm, makes a passage more engaging, and gives writers an opportunity to demonstrate their writing style. Writing that uses the same length or type of sentence without variation can be boring or difficult to read. To evaluate a passage for effective sentence variety, it is helpful to note whether the passage contains diverse sentence structures and lengths. It is also important to pay attention to the way each sentence starts and avoid beginning with the same words or phrases.

Sentence Fragments

Recall that a group of words must contain at least one **independent clause** in order to be considered a sentence. If it doesn't contain even one independent clause, it is called a **sentence fragment**.

The appropriate process for **repairing** a sentence fragment depends on what type of fragment it is. If the fragment is a dependent clause, it can sometimes be as simple as removing a subordinating word (e.g., when, because, if) from the beginning of the fragment. Alternatively, a dependent clause can be incorporated into a closely related neighboring sentence. If the fragment is missing some required part, like a subject or a verb, the fix might be as simple as adding the missing part.

Examples:

Fragment: Because he wanted to sail the Mediterranean.

Removed subordinating word: He wanted to sail the Mediterranean.

Combined with another sentence: Because he wanted to sail the Mediterranean, he booked a Greek island cruise.

Run-on Sentences

Run-on sentences consist of multiple independent clauses that have not been joined together properly. Run-on sentences can be corrected in several different ways:

Join clauses properly: This can be done with a comma and coordinating conjunction, with a semicolon, or with a colon or dash if the second clause is explaining something in the first.

Example:

> **Incorrect**: I went on the trip, we visited lots of castles.
>
> **Corrected**: I went on the trip, and we visited lots of castles.

Split into separate sentences: This correction is most effective when the independent clauses are very long or when they are not closely related.

Example:

> **Incorrect**: The drive to New York takes ten hours, my uncle lives in Boston.
>
> **Corrected**: The drive to New York takes ten hours. My uncle lives in Boston.

Make one clause dependent: This is the easiest way to make the sentence correct and more interesting at the same time. It's often as simple as adding a subordinating word between the two clauses or before the first clause.

Example:

> **Incorrect**: I finally made it to the store and I bought some eggs.
>
> **Corrected**: When I finally made it to the store, I bought some eggs.

Reduce to one clause with a compound verb: If both clauses have the same subject, remove the subject from the second clause, and you now have just one clause with a compound verb.

Example:

> **Incorrect**: The drive to New York takes ten hours, it makes me very tired.
>
> **Corrected**: The drive to New York takes ten hours and makes me very tired.

Note: While these are the simplest ways to correct a run-on sentence, often the best way is to completely reorganize the thoughts in the sentence and rewrite it.

Review Video: Fragments and Run-on Sentences
Visit mometrix.com/academy and enter code: 541989

Dangling and Misplaced Modifiers

Dangling Modifiers

A dangling modifier is a dependent clause or verbal phrase that does not have a clear logical connection to a word in the sentence.

Example:

dangling modifier

Incorrect: Reading each magazine article, the stories caught my attention.

The word *stories* cannot be modified by *Reading each magazine article*. People can read, but stories cannot read. Therefore, the subject of the sentence must be a person.

gerund phrase

Corrected: Reading each magazine article, I was entertained by the stories.

Example:

dangling modifier

Incorrect: Ever since childhood, my grandparents have visited me for Christmas.

The speaker in this sentence can't have been visited by her grandparents when *they* were children, since she wouldn't have been born yet. Either the modifier should be clarified or the sentence should be rearranged to specify whose childhood is being referenced.

dependent clause

Clarified: Ever since I was a child, my grandparents have visited for Christmas.

adverb phrase

Rearranged: Ever since childhood, I have enjoyed my grandparents visiting for Christmas.

Misplaced Modifiers

Because modifiers are grammatically versatile, they can be put in many different places within the structure of a sentence. The danger of this versatility is that a modifier can accidentally be placed where it is modifying the wrong word or where it is not clear which word it is modifying.

Example:

modifier

Incorrect: She read the book to a crowd that was filled with beautiful pictures.

The book was filled with beautiful pictures, not the crowd.

modifier

Corrected: She read the book that was filled with beautiful pictures to a crowd.

Example:

modifier

Ambiguous: Derek saw a bus nearly hit a man on his way to work.

Was Derek on his way to work or was the other man?

modifier

Derek: On his way to work, Derek saw a bus nearly hit a man.

modifier

The other man: Derek saw a bus nearly hit a man who was on his way to work.

SPLIT INFINITIVES

A split infinitive occurs when a modifying word comes between the word *to* and the verb that pairs with *to*.

Example: To *clearly* explain vs. *To explain* clearly | To *softly* sing vs. *To sing* softly

Though considered improper by some, split infinitives may provide better clarity and simplicity in some cases than the alternatives. As such, avoiding them should not be considered a universal rule.

DOUBLE NEGATIVES

Standard English allows **two negatives** only when a **positive** meaning is intended. (e.g., The team was *not displeased* with their performance.) Double negatives to emphasize negation are not used in standard English.

Negative modifiers (e.g., never, no, and not) should not be paired with other negative modifiers or negative words (e.g., none, nobody, nothing, or neither). The modifiers *hardly, barely*, and *scarcely* are also considered negatives in standard English, so they should not be used with other negatives.

Punctuation

END PUNCTUATION

PERIODS

Use a period to end all sentences except direct questions and exclamations. Periods are also used for abbreviations.

Examples: 3 p.m. | 2 a.m. | Mr. Jones | Mrs. Stevens | Dr. Smith | Bill, Jr. | Pennsylvania Ave.

Note: An abbreviation is a shortened form of a word or phrase.

Question Marks

Question marks should be used following a **direct question**. A polite request can be followed by a period instead of a question mark.

Direct Question: What is for lunch today? | How are you? | Why is that the answer?

Polite Requests: Can you please send me the item tomorrow. | Will you please walk with me on the track.

Review Video: Question Marks
Visit mometrix.com/academy and enter code: 118471

Exclamation Marks

Exclamation marks are used after a word group or sentence that shows much feeling or has special importance. Exclamation marks should not be overused. They are saved for proper **exclamatory interjections**.

Example: We're going to the finals! | You have a beautiful car! | "That's crazy!" she yelled.

Review Video: Exclamation Points
Visit mometrix.com/academy and enter code: 199367

Commas

The comma is a punctuation mark that can help you understand connections in a sentence. Not every sentence needs a comma. However, if a sentence needs a comma, you need to put it in the right place. A comma in the wrong place (or an absent comma) will make a sentence's meaning unclear.

These are some of the rules for commas:

Use Case	Example
Before a **coordinating conjunction** joining independent clauses	Bob caught three fish, and I caught two fish.
After an **introductory phrase**	After the final out, we went to a restaurant to celebrate.
After an **adverbial clause**	Studying the stars, I was awed by the beauty of the sky.
Between **items in a series**	I will bring the turkey, the pie, and the coffee.
For **interjections**	Wow, you know how to play this game.
After ***yes*** **and** ***no*** **responses**	No, I cannot come tomorrow.
Separate **nonessential modifiers**	John Frank, who coaches the team, was promoted today.
Separate **nonessential appositives**	Thomas Edison, an American inventor, was born in Ohio.
Separate **nouns of direct address**	You, John, are my only hope in this moment.
Separate **interrogative tags**	This is the last time, correct?
Separate **contrasts**	You are my friend, not my enemy.
Writing **dates**	July 4, 1776, is an important date to remember.
Writing **addresses**	He is meeting me at 456 Delaware Avenue, Washington, D.C., tomorrow morning.
Writing **geographical names**	Paris, France, is my favorite city.
Writing **titles**	John Smith, PhD, will be visiting your class today.
Separate **expressions like** ***he said***	"You can start," she said, "with an apology."

A comma is also used **between coordinate adjectives** not joined with *and*. However, not all adjectives are coordinate (i.e., equal or parallel). To determine if your adjectives are coordinate, try connecting them with *and* or reversing their order. If it still sounds right, they are coordinate.

Incorrect: The kind, brown dog followed me home.

Correct: The kind, loyal dog followed me home.

Review Video: When to Use a Comma
Visit mometrix.com/academy and enter code: 786797

SEMICOLONS

The semicolon is used to join closely related independent clauses without the need for a coordinating conjunction. Semicolons are also used in place of commas to separate list elements that have internal commas. Some rules for semicolons include:

Use Case	Example
Between closely connected independent clauses **not connected with a coordinating conjunction**	You are right; we should go with your plan.
Between independent clauses **linked with a transitional word**	I think that we can agree on this; however, I am not sure about my friends.
Between items in a **series that has internal punctuation**	I have visited New York, New York; Augusta, Maine; and Baltimore, Maryland.

Review Video: How to Use Semicolons
Visit mometrix.com/academy and enter code: 370605

COLONS

The colon is used to call attention to the words that follow it. When used in a sentence, a colon should only come at the **end** of a **complete sentence**. The rules for colons are as follows:

Use Case	Example
After an independent clause to **make a list**	I want to learn many languages: Spanish, German, and Italian.
For **explanations**	There is one thing that stands out on your resume: responsibility.
To give a **quote**	He started with an idea: "We are able to do more than we imagine."
After the **greeting in a formal letter**	To Whom It May Concern:
Show **hours and minutes**	It is 3:14 p.m.
Separate a **title and subtitle**	The essay is titled "America: A Short Introduction to a Modern Country."

Review Video: Using Colons
Visit mometrix.com/academy and enter code: 868673

Vocabulary, Spelling, and Grammar

PARENTHESES

Parentheses are used for additional information. Also, they can be used to put labels for letters or numbers in a series. Parentheses should be not be used very often. If they are overused, parentheses can be a distraction instead of a help.

Examples:

Extra Information: The rattlesnake (see Image 2) is a dangerous snake of North and South America.

Series: Include in the email (1) your name, (2) your address, and (3) your question for the author.

Review Video: Parentheses
Visit mometrix.com/academy and enter code: 947743

QUOTATION MARKS

Use quotation marks to close off **direct quotations** of a person's spoken or written words. Do not use quotation marks around indirect quotations. An indirect quotation gives someone's message without using the person's exact words. Use **single quotation marks** to close off a quotation inside a quotation.

Direct Quote: Nancy said, "I am waiting for Henry to arrive."

Indirect Quote: Henry said that he is going to be late to the meeting.

Quote inside a Quote: The teacher asked, "Has everyone read 'The Gift of the Magi'?"

Quotation marks should be used around the titles of **short works**: newspaper and magazine articles, poems, short stories, songs, television episodes, radio programs, and subdivisions of books or websites.

Examples:

"Rip Van Winkle" (short story by Washington Irving)

"O Captain! My Captain!" (poem by Walt Whitman)

Although it is not standard usage, quotation marks are sometimes used to highlight **irony** or the use of words to mean something other than their dictionary definition. This type of usage should be employed sparingly, if at all.

Examples:

The boss warned Frank that he was walking on "thin ice."	Frank is not walking on real ice. Instead, he is being warned to avoid mistakes.
The teacher thanked the young man for his "honesty."	The quotation marks around *honesty* show that the teacher does not believe the young man's explanation.

Review Video: Quotation Marks
Visit mometrix.com/academy and enter code: 884918

Periods and commas are put **inside** quotation marks. Colons and semicolons are put **outside** the quotation marks. Question marks and exclamation points are placed inside quotation marks when they are part of a quote. When the question or exclamation mark goes with the whole sentence, the mark is left outside of the quotation marks.

Examples:

Period and comma	We read "The Gift of the Magi," "The Skylight Room," and "The Cactus."
Semicolon	They watched "The Nutcracker"; then, they went home.
Exclamation mark that is a part of a quote	The crowd cheered, "Victory!"
Question mark that goes with the whole sentence	Is your favorite short story "The Tell-Tale Heart"?

APOSTROPHES

An apostrophe is used to show **possession** or the **deletion of letters in contractions**. An apostrophe is not needed with the possessive pronouns *his, hers, its, ours, theirs, whose*, and *yours*.

Singular Nouns: David's car | a book's theme | my brother's board game

Plural Nouns that end with -*s*: the scissors' handle | boys' basketball

Plural Nouns that end without -*s*: Men's department | the people's adventure

Review Video: When to Use an Apostrophe
Visit mometrix.com/academy and enter code: 213068

Review Video: Punctuation Errors in Possessive Pronouns
Visit mometrix.com/academy and enter code: 221438

HYPHENS

Hyphens are used to **separate compound words**. Use hyphens in the following cases:

Use Case	Example
Compound numbers from 21 to 99 when written out in words	This team needs twenty-five points to win the game.
Written-out fractions that are used as adjectives	The recipe says that we need a three-fourths cup of butter.
Compound adjectives that come before a noun	The well-fed dog took a nap.
Unusual compound words that would be hard to read or easily confused with other words	This is the best anti-itch cream on the market.

Note: This is not a complete set of the rules for hyphens. A dictionary is the best tool for knowing if a compound word needs a hyphen.

Review Video: Hyphens
Visit mometrix.com/academy and enter code: 981632

Dashes

Dashes are used to show a **break** or a **change in thought** in a sentence or to act as parentheses in a sentence. When typing, use two hyphens to make a dash. Do not put a space before or after the dash. The following are the functions of dashes:

Use Case	Example
Set off parenthetical statements or an **appositive with internal punctuation**	The three trees—oak, pine, and magnolia—are coming on a truck tomorrow.
Show a **break or change in tone or thought**	The first question—how silly of me—does not have a correct answer.

Ellipsis Marks

The ellipsis mark has **three** periods (…) to show when **words have been removed** from a quotation. If a **full sentence or more** is removed from a quoted passage, you need to use **four** periods to show the removed text and the end punctuation mark. The ellipsis mark should not be used at the beginning of a quotation. The ellipsis mark should also not be used at the end of a quotation unless some words have been deleted from the end of the final quoted sentence.

Example:

> "Then he picked up the groceries...paid for them...later he went home."

Brackets

There are two main reasons to use brackets:

Use Case	Example
Placing **parentheses inside of parentheses**	The hero of this story, Paul Revere (a silversmith and industrialist [see Ch. 4]), rode through towns of Massachusetts to warn of advancing British troops.
Adding **clarification or detail to a quotation** that is not part of the quotation	The father explained, "My children are planning to attend my alma mater [State University]."

Review Video: Brackets
Visit mometrix.com/academy and enter code: 727546

Common Usage Mistakes

Word Confusion

Which, That, and Who

The words *which*, *that*, and *who* can act as **relative pronouns** to help clarify or describe a noun.

Which is used for things only.

> Example: Andrew's car, *which is old and rusty,* broke down last week.

That is used for people or things. *That* is usually informal when used to describe people.

> Example: Is this the only book *that Louis L'Amour wrote?*

> Example: Is Louis L'Amour the author *that wrote Western novels?*

Who is used for people or for animals that have an identity or personality.

> Example: Mozart was the composer *who wrote those operas.*

> Example: John's dog, *who is called Max,* is large and fierce.

Homophones

Homophones are words that sound alike (or similar) but have different **spellings** and **definitions**. A homophone is a type of **homonym**, which is a pair or group of words that are pronounced or spelled the same, but do not mean the same thing.

To, Too, and Two

To can be an adverb or a preposition for showing direction, purpose, and relationship. See your dictionary for the many other ways to use *to* in a sentence.

> Examples: I went to the store. | I want to go with you.

Too is an adverb that means *also, as well, very,* or *in excess.*

> Examples: I can walk a mile too. | You have eaten too much.

Two is a number.

> Example: You have two minutes left.

There, Their, and They're

There can be an adjective, adverb, or pronoun. Often, *there* is used to show a place or to start a sentence.

> Examples: I went there yesterday. | There is something in his pocket.

Their is a pronoun that is used to show ownership.

> Examples: He is their father. | This is their fourth apology this week.

They're is a contraction of *they are.*

> Example: Did you know that they're in town?

Vocabulary, Spelling, and Grammar

Knew and New

Knew is the past tense of *know.*

Example: I knew the answer.

New is an adjective that means something is current, has not been used, or is modern.

Example: This is my new phone.

Then and Than

Then is an adverb that indicates sequence or order:

Example: I'm going to run to the library and then come home.

Than is special-purpose word used only for comparisons:

Example: Susie likes chips more than candy.

Its and It's

Its is a pronoun that shows ownership.

Example: The guitar is in its case.

It's is a contraction of *it is.*

Example: It's an honor and a privilege to meet you.

Note: The *h* in honor is silent, so *honor* starts with the vowel sound *o*, which must have the article *an*.

Your and You're

Your is a pronoun that shows ownership.

Example: This is your moment to shine.

You're is a contraction of *you are.*

Example: Yes, you're correct.

Saw and Seen

Saw is the past-tense form of *see.*

Example: I saw a turtle on my walk this morning.

Seen is the past participle of *see.*

Example: I have seen this movie before.

Affect and Effect

There are two main reasons that *affect* and *effect* are so often confused: 1) both words can be used as either a noun or a verb, and 2) unlike most homophones, their usage and meanings are closely related to each other. Here is a quick rundown of the four usage options:

Affect (n): feeling, emotion, or mood that is displayed

Example: The patient had a flat *affect.* (i.e., his face showed little or no emotion)

Affect (v): to alter, to change, to influence

Example: The sunshine *affects* the plant's growth.

Effect (n): a result, a consequence

Example: What *effect* will this weather have on our schedule?

Effect (v): to bring about, to cause to be

Example: These new rules will *effect* order in the office.

The noun form of *affect* is rarely used outside of technical medical descriptions, so if a noun form is needed on the test, you can safely select *effect.* The verb form of *effect* is not as rare as the noun form of *affect,* but it's still not all that likely to show up on your test. If you need a verb and you can't decide which to use based on the definitions, choosing *affect* is your best bet.

Homographs

Homographs are words that share the same spelling, but have different meanings and sometimes different pronunciations. To figure out which meaning is being used, you should be looking for context clues. The context clues give hints to the meaning of the word. For example, the word *spot* has many meanings. It can mean "a place" or "a stain or blot." In the sentence "After my lunch, I saw a spot on my shirt," the word *spot* means "a stain or blot." The context clues of "After my lunch" and "on my shirt" guide you to this decision. A homograph is another type of homonym.

Bank

(noun): an establishment where money is held for savings or lending

(verb): to collect or pile up

Content

(noun): the topics that will be addressed within a book

(adjective): pleased or satisfied

(verb): to make someone pleased or satisfied

Fine

(noun): an amount of money that acts a penalty for an offense

(adjective): very small or thin

(adverb): in an acceptable way

(verb): to make someone pay money as a punishment

Incense

(noun): a material that is burned in religious settings and makes a pleasant aroma

(verb): to frustrate or anger

LEAD

(noun): the first or highest position

(noun): a heavy metallic element

(verb): to direct a person or group of followers

(adjective): containing lead

OBJECT

(noun): a lifeless item that can be held and observed

(verb): to disagree

PRODUCE

(noun): fruits and vegetables

(verb): to make or create something

REFUSE

(noun): garbage or debris that has been thrown away

(verb): to not allow

SUBJECT

(noun): an area of study

(verb): to force or subdue

TEAR

(noun): a fluid secreted by the eyes

(verb): to separate or pull apart

COMMONLY MISUSED WORDS AND PHRASES

A LOT

The phrase *a lot* should always be written as two words; never as *alot*.

Correct: That's a lot of chocolate!

Incorrect: He does that alot.

CAN

The word *can* is used to describe things that are possible occurrences; the word *may* is used to described things that are allowed to happen.

Correct: May I have another piece of pie?

Correct: I can lift three of these bags of mulch at a time.

Incorrect: Mom said we can stay up thirty minutes later tonight.

COULD HAVE

The phrase *could of* is often incorrectly substituted for the phrase *could have*. Similarly, *could of*, *may of*, and *might of* are sometimes used in place of the correct phrases *could have*, *may have*, and *might have*.

> **Correct**: If I had known, I would have helped out.
>
> **Incorrect**: Well, that could of gone much worse than it did.

MYSELF

The word *myself* is a reflexive pronoun, often incorrectly used in place of *I* or *me*.

> **Correct**: He let me do it myself.
>
> **Incorrect**: The job was given to Dave and myself.

OFF

The phrase *off of* is a redundant expression that should be avoided. In most cases, it can be corrected simply by removing *of*.

> **Correct**: My dog chased the squirrel off its perch on the fence.
>
> **Incorrect**: He finally moved his plate off of the table.

SUPPOSED TO

The phrase *suppose to* is sometimes used incorrectly in place of the phrase *supposed to*.

> **Correct**: I was supposed to go to the store this afternoon.
>
> **Incorrect**: When are we suppose to get our grades?

TRY TO

The phrase *try and* is often used in informal writing and conversation to replace the correct phrase *try to*.

> **Correct**: It's a good policy to try to satisfy every customer who walks in the door.
>
> **Incorrect**: Don't try and do too much.

Spelling Conventions

GENERAL SPELLING RULES

WORDS ENDING WITH A CONSONANT

Usually, the final consonant is **doubled** on a word before adding a suffix. This is the rule for single syllable words, words ending with one consonant, and multi-syllable words with the last syllable accented. The following are examples:

- *beg* becomes *begging* (single syllable)
- *shop* becomes *shopped* (single syllable)
- *add* becomes *adding* (already ends in double consonant, do not add another *d*)
- *deter* becomes *deterring* (multi-syllable, accent on last syllable)

- *regret* becomes *regrettable* (multi-syllable, accent on last syllable)
- *compost* becomes *composting* (do not add another *t* because the accent is on the first syllable)

Words Ending with Y or C

The general rule for words ending in *y* is to keep the *y* when adding a suffix if the **y is preceded by a vowel**. If the word **ends in a consonant and y** the *y* is changed to an *i* before the suffix is added (unless the suffix itself begins with *i*). The following are examples:

- *pay* becomes *paying* (keep the *y*)
- *bully* becomes *bullied* (change to *i*)
- *bully* becomes *bullying* (keep the *y* because the suffix is *–ing*)

If a word ends with *c* and the suffix begins with an *e, i,* or *y*, the letter *k* is usually added to the end of the word. The following are examples:

- panic becomes panicky
- mimic becomes mimicking

Words Containing IE or EI, and/or Ending with E

Most words are spelled with an *i* before *e*, except when they follow the letter *c*, **or** sound like *a*. For example, the following words are spelled correctly according to these rules:

- piece, friend, believe (*i* before *e*)
- receive, ceiling, conceited (except after *c*)
- weight, neighborhood, veil (sounds like *a*)

To add a suffix to words ending with the letter *e*, first determine if the *e* is silent. If it is, the *e* will be kept if the added suffix begins with a consonant. If the suffix begins with a vowel, the *e* is dropped. The following are examples:

- *age* becomes *ageless* (keep the *e*)
- *age* becomes *aging* (drop the *e*)

An exception to this rule occurs when the word ends in *ce* or *ge* and the suffix *able* or *ous* is added; these words will retain the letter *e*. The following are examples:

- courage becomes courageous
- notice becomes noticeable

Words Ending with ISE or IZE

A small number of words end with *ise*. Most of the words in the English language with the same sound end in *ize*. The following are examples:

- advertise, advise, arise, chastise, circumcise, and comprise
- compromise, demise, despise, devise, disguise, enterprise, excise, and exercise
- franchise, improvise, incise, merchandise, premise, reprise, and revise
- supervise, surmise, surprise, and televise

Words that end with *ize* include the following:

- accessorize, agonize, authorize, and brutalize
- capitalize, caramelize, categorize, civilize, and demonize
- downsize, empathize, euthanize, idolize, and immunize
- legalize, metabolize, mobilize, organize, and ostracize
- plagiarize, privatize, utilize, and visualize

(Note that some words may technically be spelled with *ise*, especially in British English, but it is more common to use *ize*. Examples include *symbolize/symbolise* and *baptize/baptise*.)

WORDS ENDING WITH CEED, SEDE, OR CEDE

There are only three words in the English language that end with *ceed*: *exceed, proceed,* and *succeed*. There is only one word in the English language that ends with *sede*: *supersede*. Most other words that sound like *sede* or *ceed* end with *cede*. The following are examples:

- concede, recede, and precede

WORDS ENDING IN ABLE OR IBLE

For words ending in *able* or *ible*, there are no hard and fast rules. The following are examples:

- adjustable, unbeatable, collectable, deliverable, and likeable
- edible, compatible, feasible, sensible, and credible

There are more words ending in *able* than *ible*; this is useful to know if guessing is necessary.

WORDS ENDING IN ANCE OR ENCE

The suffixes *ence, ency,* and *ent* are used in the following cases:

- the suffix is preceded by the letter *c* but sounds like *s* – *innocence*
- the suffix is preceded by the letter *g* but sounds like *j* – *intelligence, negligence*

The suffixes *ance, ancy,* and *ant* are used in the following cases:

- the suffix is preceded by the letter *c* but sounds like *k* – *significant, vacant*
- the suffix is preceded by the letter *g* with a hard sound – *elegant, extravagance*

If the suffix is preceded by other letters, there are no clear rules. For example: *finance, abundance,* and *assistance* use the letter *a,* while *decadence, competence,* and *excellence* use the letter *e*.

WORDS ENDING IN TION, SION, OR CIAN

Words ending in *tion, sion,* or *cian* all sound like *shun* or *zhun*. There are no rules for which ending is used for words. The following are examples:

- action, agitation, caution, fiction, nation, and motion
- admission, expression, mansion, permission, and television
- electrician, magician, musician, optician, and physician (note that these words tend to describe occupations)

Words with the AI or IA Combination

When deciding if *ai* or *ia* is correct, the combination of *ai* usually sounds like one vowel sound, as in *Britain*, while the vowels in *ia* are pronounced separately, as in *guardian*. The following are examples:

- captain, certain, faint, hair, malaise, and praise (*ai* makes one sound)
- bacteria, beneficiary, diamond, humiliation, and nuptial (*ia* makes two sounds)

Rules for Plurals

Nouns Ending in CH, SH, S, X, or Z

When a noun ends in the letters *ch, sh, s, x,* or *z*, an *es* instead of a singular *s* is added to the end of the word to make it plural. The following are examples:

- church becomes churches
- bush becomes bushes
- bass becomes basses
- mix becomes mixes
- buzz becomes buzzes

This is the rule with proper names as well; the Ross family would become the Rosses.

Nouns Ending in Y or AY/EY/IY/OY/UY

If a noun ends with a **consonant and y**, the plural is formed by replacing the *y* with *ies*. For example, *fly* becomes *flies* and *puppy* becomes *puppies*. If a noun ends with a **vowel and *y***, the plural is formed by adding an *s*. For example, *alley* becomes *alleys* and *boy* becomes *boys*.

Nouns Ending in F or FE

Most nouns ending in *f* or *fe* are pluralized by replacing the *f* with *v* and adding *es*. The following are examples:

- knife becomes knives; self becomes selves; wolf becomes wolves.

An exception to this rule is the word *roof; roof* becomes *roofs*.

Nouns Ending in O

Most nouns ending with a **consonant and *o*** are pluralized by adding *es*. The following are examples:

- hero becomes heroes; tornado becomes tornadoes; potato becomes potatoes

Most nouns ending with a **vowel and *o*** are pluralized by adding *s*. The following are examples:

- portfolio becomes portfolios; radio becomes radios; cameo becomes cameos.

An exception to these rules is seen with musical terms ending in *o*. These words are pluralized by adding *s* even if they end in a consonant and *o*. The following are examples: *soprano* becomes *sopranos; banjo* becomes *banjos; piano* becomes *pianos.*

Letters, Numbers, and Symbols

Letters and numbers become plural by adding an apostrophe and *s*. The following are examples:

- The *L's* are the people whose names begin with the letter *L*.
- They broke the teams down into groups of *3's*.
- The sorority girls were all *KD's*.

Compound Nouns

A **compound noun** is a noun that is made up of two or more words; they can be written with hyphens. For example, *mother-in-law* or *court-martial* are compound nouns. To make them plural, an *s* or *es* is added to the noun portion of the word. The following are examples: *mother-in-law* becomes *mothers-in-law; court-martial* becomes *courts-martial.*

Exceptions

Some words do not fall into any specific category for making the singular form plural. They are **irregular**. Certain words become plural by changing the vowels within the word. The following are examples:

- woman becomes women; goose becomes geese; foot becomes feet

Some words change in unusual ways in the plural form. The following are examples:

- mouse becomes mice; ox becomes oxen; person becomes people

Some words are the same in both the singular and plural forms. The following are examples:

- *Salmon*, *deer*, and *moose* are the same whether singular or plural.

Commonly Misspelled Words

accidentally	accommodate	accompanied	accompany
achieved	acknowledgment	across	address
aggravate	aisle	ancient	anxiety
apparently	appearance	arctic	argument
arrangement	attendance	auxiliary	awkward
bachelor	barbarian	beggar	beneficiary
biscuit	brilliant	business	cafeteria
calendar	campaign	candidate	ceiling
cemetery	changeable	changing	characteristic
chauffeur	colonel	column	commit
committee	comparative	compel	competent
competition	conceive	congratulations	conqueror
conscious	coolly	correspondent	courtesy
curiosity	cylinder	deceive	deference
deferred	definite	describe	desirable
desperate	develop	diphtheria	disappear
disappoint	disastrous	discipline	discussion
disease	dissatisfied	dissipate	drudgery
ecstasy	efficient	eighth	eligible
embarrass	emphasize	especially	exaggerate
exceed	exhaust	exhilaration	existence
explanation	extraordinary	familiar	fascinate

Vocabulary, Spelling, and Grammar

February	fiery	finally	forehead
foreign	foreigner	foremost	forfeit
ghost	glamorous	government	grammar
grateful	grief	grievous	handkerchief
harass	height	hoping	hurriedly
hygiene	hypocrisy	imminent	incidentally
incredible	independent	indigestible	inevitable
innocence	intelligible	intentionally	intercede
interest	irresistible	judgment	legitimate
liable	library	likelihood	literature
maintenance	maneuver	manual	mathematics
mattress	miniature	mischievous	misspell
momentous	mortgage	neither	nickel
niece	ninety	noticeable	notoriety
obedience	obstacle	occasion	occurrence
omitted	operate	optimistic	organization
outrageous	pageant	pamphlet	parallel
parliament	permissible	perseverance	persuade
physically	physician	possess	possibly
practically	prairie	preceding	prejudice
prevalent	professor	pronunciation	pronouncement
propeller	protein	psychiatrist	psychology
quantity	questionnaire	rally	recede
receive	recognize	recommend	referral
referred	relieve	religious	resistance
restaurant	rhetoric	rhythm	ridiculous
sacrilegious	salary	scarcely	schedule
secretary	sentinel	separate	severely
sheriff	shriek	similar	soliloquy
sophomore	species	strenuous	studying
suffrage	supersede	suppress	surprise
symmetry	temperament	temperature	tendency
tournament	tragedy	transferred	truly
twelfth	tyranny	unanimous	unpleasant
usage	vacuum	valuable	vein
vengeance	vigilance	villain	Wednesday
weird	wholly		

Word Roots and Prefixes and Suffixes

AFFIXES

Affixes in the English language are morphemes that are added to words to create related but different words. Derivational affixes form new words based on and related to the original words. For example, the affix *–ness* added to the end of the adjective *happy* forms the noun *happiness.* Inflectional affixes form different grammatical versions of words. For example, the plural affix *–s* changes the singular noun *book* to the plural noun *books*, and the past tense affix *–ed* changes the present tense verb *look* to the past tense *looked.* Prefixes are affixes placed in front of words. For example, *heat* means to make hot; *preheat* means to heat in advance. Suffixes are affixes placed at the ends of words. The *happiness* example above contains the suffix *–ness.* Circumfixes add parts both before and after words, such as how *light* becomes *enlighten* with the prefix *en-* and the suffix *–en.* Interfixes create compound words via central affixes: *speed* and *meter* become *speedometer* via the interfix *–o–*.

Review Video: Affixes
Visit mometrix.com/academy and enter code: 782422

WORD ROOTS, PREFIXES, AND SUFFIXES TO HELP DETERMINE MEANINGS OF WORDS

Many English words were formed from combining multiple sources. For example, the Latin *habēre* means "to have," and the prefixes *in-* and *im-* mean a lack or prevention of something, as in *insufficient* and *imperfect.* Latin combined *in-* with *habēre* to form *inhibēre,* whose past participle was *inhibitus*. This is the origin of the English word *inhibit,* meaning to prevent from having. Hence by knowing the meanings of both the prefix and the root, one can decipher the word meaning. In Greek, the root *enkephalo-* refers to the brain. Many medical terms are based on this root, such as encephalitis and hydrocephalus. Understanding the prefix and suffix meanings (*-itis* means inflammation; *hydro-* means water) allows a person to deduce that encephalitis refers to brain inflammation and hydrocephalus refers to water (or other fluid) in the brain.

Review Video: Root Words in English
Visit mometrix.com/academy and enter code: 896380

Review Video: Determining Word Meanings
Visit mometrix.com/academy and enter code: 894894

PREFIXES

Knowing common prefixes is helpful for all readers as they try to determining meanings or definitions of unfamiliar words. For example, a common word used when cooking is *preheat.* Knowing that *pre-* means in advance can also inform them that *presume* means to assume in advance, that *prejudice* means advance judgment, and that this understanding can be applied to many other words beginning with *pre-*. Knowing that the prefix *dis-* indicates opposition informs the meanings of words like *disbar, disagree, disestablish,* and many more. Knowing *dys-* means bad, impaired, abnormal, or difficult informs *dyslogistic, dysfunctional, dysphagia,* and *dysplasia.*

SUFFIXES

In English, certain suffixes generally indicate both that a word is a noun, and that the noun represents a state of being or quality. For example, *-ness* is commonly used to change an adjective into its noun form, as with *happy* and *happiness, nice* and *niceness,* and so on. The suffix *–tion* is commonly used to transform a verb into its noun form, as with *converse* and *conversation or move* and *motion*. Thus, if readers are unfamiliar with the second form of a word, knowing the meaning of the transforming suffix can help them determine meaning.

Prefixes for Numbers

Prefix	Definition	Examples
bi-	two	bisect, biennial
mono-	one, single	monogamy, monologue
poly-	many	polymorphous, polygamous
semi-	half, partly	semicircle, semicolon
uni-	one	uniform, unity

Prefixes for Time, Direction, and Space

Prefix	Definition	Examples
a-	in, on, of, up, to	abed, afoot
ab-	from, away, off	abdicate, abjure
ad-	to, toward	advance, adventure
ante-	before, previous	antecedent, antedate
anti-	against, opposing	antipathy, antidote
cata-	down, away, thoroughly	catastrophe, cataclysm
circum-	around	circumspect, circumference
com-	with, together, very	commotion, complicate
contra-	against, opposing	contradict, contravene
de-	from	depart
dia-	through, across, apart	diameter, diagnose
dis-	away, off, down, not	dissent, disappear
epi-	upon	epilogue
ex-	out	extract, excerpt
hypo-	under, beneath	hypodermic, hypothesis
inter-	among, between	intercede, interrupt
intra-	within	intramural, intrastate
ob-	against, opposing	objection
per-	through	perceive, permit
peri-	around	periscope, perimeter
post-	after, following	postpone, postscript
pre-	before, previous	prevent, preclude
pro-	forward, in place of	propel, pronoun
retro-	back, backward	retrospect, retrograde
sub-	under, beneath	subjugate, substitute
super-	above, extra	supersede, supernumerary
trans-	across, beyond, over	transact, transport
ultra-	beyond, excessively	ultramodern, ultrasonic

Negative Prefixes

Prefix	Definition	Examples
a-	without, lacking	atheist, agnostic
in-	not, opposing	incapable, ineligible
non-	not	nonentity, nonsense
un-	not, reverse of	unhappy, unlock

EXTRA PREFIXES

Prefix	Definition	Examples
for-	away, off, from	forget, forswear
fore-	previous	foretell, forefathers
homo-	same, equal	homogenized, homonym
hyper-	excessive, over	hypercritical, hypertension
in-	in, into	intrude, invade
mal-	bad, poorly, not	malfunction, malpractice
mis-	bad, poorly, not	misspell, misfire
neo-	new	Neolithic, neoconservative
omni-	all, everywhere	omniscient, omnivore
ortho-	right, straight	orthogonal, orthodox
over-	above	overbearing, oversight
pan-	all, entire	panorama, pandemonium
para-	beside, beyond	parallel, paradox
re-	backward, again	revoke, recur
sym-	with, together	sympathy, symphony

Below is a list of common suffixes and their meanings:

ADJECTIVE SUFFIXES

Suffix	Definition	Examples
-able (-ible)	capable of being	toler*able*, ed*ible*
-esque	in the style of, like	picturesque, grotesque
-ful	filled with, marked by	thankful, zestful
-ific	make, cause	terrific, beatific
-ish	suggesting, like	churlish, childish
-less	lacking, without	hopeless, countless
-ous	marked by, given to	religious, riotous

NOUN SUFFIXES

Suffix	Definition	Examples
-acy	state, condition	accuracy, privacy
-ance	act, condition, fact	acceptance, vigilance
-ard	one that does excessively	drunkard, sluggard
-ation	action, state, result	occupation, starvation
-dom	state, rank, condition	serfdom, wisdom
-er (-or)	office, action	teach*er*, elevat*or*, hon*or*
-ess	feminine	waitress, duchess
-hood	state, condition	manhood, statehood
-ion	action, result, state	union, fusion
-ism	act, manner, doctrine	barbarism, socialism
-ist	worker, follower	monopolist, socialist
-ity (-ty)	state, quality, condition	acid*ity*, civil*ity*, twen*ty*
-ment	result, action	Refreshment
-ness	quality, state	greatness, tallness
-ship	position	internship, statesmanship
-sion (-tion)	state, result	revi*sion*, expedi*tion*
-th	act, state, quality	warmth, width

Suffix	Definition	Examples
-tude	quality, state, result	magnitude, fortitude

Verb Suffixes

Suffix	Definition	Examples
-ate	having, showing	separate, desolate
-en	cause to be, become	deepen, strengthen
-fy	make, cause to have	glorify, fortify
-ize	cause to be, treat with	sterilize, mechanize

Nuance and Word Meanings

Synonyms and Antonyms

When you understand how words relate to each other, you will discover more in a passage. This is explained by understanding **synonyms** (e.g., words that mean the same thing) and **antonyms** (e.g., words that mean the opposite of one another). As an example, *dry* and *arid* are synonyms, and *dry* and *wet* are antonyms.

There are many pairs of words in English that can be considered synonyms, despite having slightly different definitions. For instance, the words *friendly* and *collegial* can both be used to describe a warm interpersonal relationship, and one would be correct to call them synonyms. However, *collegial* (kin to *colleague*) is often used in reference to professional or academic relationships, and *friendly* has no such connotation.

If the difference between the two words is too great, then they should not be called synonyms. *Hot* and *warm* are not synonyms because their meanings are too distinct. A good way to determine whether two words are synonyms is to substitute one word for the other word and verify that the meaning of the sentence has not changed. Substituting *warm* for *hot* in a sentence would convey a different meaning. Although warm and hot may seem close in meaning, warm generally means that the temperature is moderate, and hot generally means that the temperature is excessively high.

Antonyms are words with opposite meanings. *Light* and *dark*, *up* and *down*, *right* and *left*, *good* and *bad*: these are all sets of antonyms. Be careful to distinguish between antonyms and pairs of words that are simply different. *Black* and *gray*, for instance, are not antonyms because gray is not the opposite of black. *Black* and *white*, on the other hand, are antonyms.

Not every word has an antonym. For instance, many nouns do not. What would be the antonym of *chair*? During your exam, the questions related to antonyms are more likely to concern adjectives. You will recall that adjectives are words that describe a noun. Some common adjectives include *purple*, *fast*, *skinny*, and *sweet*. From those four adjectives, *purple* is the item that lacks a group of obvious antonyms.

Review Video: Synonyms and Antonyms
Visit mometrix.com/academy and enter code: 105612

Denotative vs. Connotative Meaning

The **denotative** meaning of a word is the literal meaning. The **connotative** meaning goes beyond the denotative meaning to include the emotional reaction that a word may invoke. The connotative meaning often takes the denotative meaning a step further due to associations the reader makes with the denotative meaning. Readers can differentiate between the denotative and connotative meanings by first recognizing how authors use each meaning. Most non-fiction, for example, is fact-based and authors do not use flowery, figurative language. The reader can assume that the writer is using the denotative meaning of words. In fiction, the author may use the connotative meaning. Readers can determine whether the author is using the denotative or connotative meaning of a word by implementing context clues.

> **Review Video: Connotation and Denotation**
> Visit mometrix.com/academy and enter code: 310092

Nuances of Word Meaning Relative to Connotation, Denotation, Diction, and Usage

A word's denotation is simply its objective dictionary definition. However, its connotation refers to the subjective associations, often emotional, that specific words evoke in listeners and readers. Two or more words can have the same dictionary meaning, but very different connotations. Writers use diction (word choice) to convey various nuances of thought and emotion by selecting synonyms for other words that best communicate the associations they want to trigger for readers. For example, a car engine is naturally greasy; in this sense, "greasy" is a neutral term. But when a person's smile, appearance, or clothing is described as "greasy," it has a negative connotation. Some words have even gained additional or different meanings over time. For example, *awful* used to be used to describe things that evoked a sense of awe. When *awful* is separated into its root word, awe, and suffix, -ful, it can be understood to mean "full of awe." However, the word is now commonly used to describe things that evoke repulsion, terror, or another intense, negative reaction.

> **Review Video: Word Usage in Sentences**
> Visit mometrix.com/academy and enter code: 197863

Using Context to Determine Meaning

Context Clues

Readers of all levels will encounter words that they have either never seen or have encountered only on a limited basis. The best way to define a word in **context** is to look for nearby words that can assist in revealing the meaning of the word. For instance, unfamiliar nouns are often accompanied by examples that provide a definition. Consider the following sentence: *Dave arrived at the party in hilarious garb: a leopard-print shirt, buckskin trousers, and bright green sneakers.* If a reader was unfamiliar with the meaning of garb, he or she could read the examples (i.e., a leopard-print shirt, buckskin trousers, and bright green sneakers) and quickly determine that the word means *clothing*. Examples will not always be this obvious. Consider this sentence: *Parsley, lemon, and flowers were just a few of the items he used as garnishes.* Here, the word *garnishes* is exemplified by parsley, lemon, and flowers. Readers who have eaten in a variety of restaurants will probably be able to identify a garnish as something used to decorate a plate.

> **Review Video: Reading Comprehension: Using Context Clues**
> Visit mometrix.com/academy and enter code: 613660

Using Contrast in Context Clues

In addition to looking at the context of a passage, readers can use contrast to define an unfamiliar word in context. In many sentences, the author will not describe the unfamiliar word directly; instead, he or she will describe the opposite of the unfamiliar word. Thus, you are provided with some information that will bring you closer to defining the word. Consider the following example:

Despite his intelligence, Hector's low brow and bad posture made him look obtuse. The author writes that Hector's appearance does not convey intelligence. Therefore, *obtuse* must mean unintelligent. Here is another example: *Despite the horrible weather, we were beatific about our trip to Alaska.* The word *despite* indicates that the speaker's feelings were at odds with the weather. Since the weather is described as *horrible*, then *beatific* must mean something positive.

Substitution to Find Meaning

In some cases, there will be very few contextual clues to help a reader define the meaning of an unfamiliar word. When this happens, one strategy that readers may employ is **substitution**. A good reader will brainstorm some possible synonyms for the given word, and he or she will substitute these words into the sentence. If the sentence and the surrounding passage continue to make sense, then the substitution has revealed at least some information about the unfamiliar word. Consider the sentence: *Frank's admonition rang in her ears as she climbed the mountain.* A reader unfamiliar with *admonition* might come up with some substitutions like *vow*, *promise*, *advice*, *complaint*, or *compliment*. All of these words make general sense of the sentence, though their meanings are diverse. However, this process has suggested that an admonition is some sort of message. The substitution strategy is rarely able to pinpoint a precise definition, but this process can be effective as a last resort.

Occasionally, you will be able to define an unfamiliar word by looking at the descriptive words in the context. Consider the following sentence: *Fred dragged the recalcitrant boy kicking and screaming up the stairs.* The words *dragged*, *kicking*, and *screaming* all suggest that the boy does not want to go up the stairs. The reader may assume that *recalcitrant* means something like unwilling or protesting. In this example, an unfamiliar adjective was identified.

Additionally, using description to define an unfamiliar noun is a common practice compared to unfamiliar adjectives, as in this sentence: *Don's wrinkled frown and constantly shaking fist identified him as a curmudgeon of the first order.* Don is described as having a *wrinkled frown and constantly shaking fist*, suggesting that a *curmudgeon* must be a grumpy person. Contrasts do not always provide detailed information about the unfamiliar word, but they at least give the reader some clues.

Words with Multiple Meanings

When a word has more than one meaning, readers can have difficulty determining how the word is being used in a given sentence. For instance, the verb *cleave*, can mean either *join* or *separate*. When readers come upon this word, they will have to select the definition that makes the most sense. Consider the following sentence: *Hermione's knife cleaved the bread cleanly.* Since a knife cannot join bread together, the word must indicate separation. A slightly more difficult example would be the sentence: *The birds cleaved to one another as they flew from the oak tree.* Immediately, the presence of the words *to one another* should suggest that in this sentence *cleave* is being used to mean *join*. Discovering the intent of a word with multiple meanings requires the same tricks as defining an unknown word: look for contextual clues and evaluate the substituted words.

Context Clues to Help Determine Meanings of Words

If readers simply bypass unknown words, they can reach unclear conclusions about what they read. However, looking for the definition of every unfamiliar word in the dictionary can slow their reading progress. Moreover, the dictionary may list multiple definitions for a word, so readers must search the word's context for meaning. Hence context is important to new vocabulary regardless of reader methods. Four types of context clues are examples, definitions, descriptive words, and opposites. Authors may use a certain word, and then follow it with several different examples of what it describes. Sometimes authors actually supply a definition of a word they use, which is especially true in informational and technical texts. Authors may use descriptive words that elaborate upon a vocabulary word they just used. Authors may also use opposites with negation that help define meaning.

EXAMPLES AND DEFINITIONS

An author may use a word and then give examples that illustrate its meaning. Consider this text: "Teachers who do not know how to use sign language can help students who are deaf or hard of hearing understand certain instructions by using gestures instead, like pointing their fingers to indicate which direction to look or go; holding up a hand, palm outward, to indicate stopping; holding the hands flat, palms up, curling a finger toward oneself in a beckoning motion to indicate 'come here'; or curling all fingers toward oneself repeatedly to indicate 'come on', 'more', or 'continue.'" The author of this text has used the word "gestures" and then followed it with examples, so a reader unfamiliar with the word could deduce from the examples that "gestures" means "hand motions." Readers can find examples by looking for signal words "for example," "for instance," "like," "such as," and "e.g."

While readers sometimes have to look for definitions of unfamiliar words in a dictionary or do some work to determine a word's meaning from its surrounding context, at other times an author may make it easier for readers by defining certain words. For example, an author may write, "The company did not have sufficient capital, that is, available money, to continue operations." The author defined "capital" as "available money," and heralded the definition with the phrase "that is." Another way that authors supply word definitions is with appositives. Rather than being introduced by a signal phrase like "that is," "namely," or "meaning," an appositive comes after the vocabulary word it defines and is enclosed within two commas. For example, an author may write, "The Indians introduced the Pilgrims to pemmican, cakes they made of lean meat dried and mixed with fat, which proved greatly beneficial to keep settlers from starving while trapping." In this example, the appositive phrase following "pemmican" and preceding "which" defines the word "pemmican."

DESCRIPTIONS

When readers encounter a word they do not recognize in a text, the author may expand on that word to illustrate it better. While the author may do this to make the prose more picturesque and vivid, the reader can also take advantage of this description to provide context clues to the meaning of the unfamiliar word. For example, an author may write, "The man sitting next to me on the airplane was obese. His shirt stretched across his vast expanse of flesh, strained almost to bursting." The descriptive second sentence elaborates on and helps to define the previous sentence's word "obese" to mean extremely fat. A reader unfamiliar with the word "repugnant" can decipher its meaning through an author's accompanying description: "The way the child grimaced and shuddered as he swallowed the medicine showed that its taste was particularly repugnant."

OPPOSITES

Text authors sometimes introduce a contrasting or opposing idea before or after a concept they present. They may do this to emphasize or heighten the idea they present by contrasting it with something that is the reverse. However, readers can also use these context clues to understand familiar words. For example, an author may write, "Our conversation was not cheery. We sat and talked very solemnly about his experience and a number of similar events." The reader who is not familiar with the word "solemnly" can deduce by the author's preceding use of "not cheery" that "solemn" means the opposite of cheery or happy, so it must mean serious or sad. Or if someone writes, "Don't condemn his entire project because you couldn't find anything good to say about it," readers unfamiliar with "condemn" can understand from the sentence structure that it means the opposite of saying anything good, so it must mean reject, dismiss, or disapprove. "Entire" adds another context clue, meaning total or complete rejection.

Syntax to Determine Part of Speech and Meanings of Words

Syntax refers to sentence structure and word order. Suppose that a reader encounters an unfamiliar word when reading a text. To illustrate, consider an invented word like "splunch." If this word is used in a sentence like "Please splunch that ball to me," the reader can assume from syntactic context that "splunch" is a verb. We would not use a noun, adjective, adverb, or preposition with the object "that ball," and the prepositional phrase "to me" further indicates "splunch" represents an action. However, in the sentence, "Please hand that splunch to me," the reader can assume that "splunch" is a noun. Demonstrative adjectives like "that" modify nouns. Also, we hand someone some*thing*—a thing being a noun; we do not hand someone a verb, adjective, or adverb. Some sentences contain further clues. For example, from the sentence, "The princess wore the glittering splunch on her head," the reader can deduce that it is a crown, tiara, or something similar from the syntactic context, without knowing the word.

Syntax to Indicate Different Meanings of Similar Sentences

The syntax, or structure, of a sentence affords grammatical cues that aid readers in comprehending the meanings of words, phrases, and sentences in the texts that they read. Seemingly minor differences in how the words or phrases in a sentence are ordered can make major differences in meaning. For example, two sentences can use exactly the same words but have different meanings based on the word order:

- "The man with a broken arm sat in a chair."
- "The man sat in a chair with a broken arm."

While both sentences indicate that a man sat in a chair, differing syntax indicates whether the man's or chair's arm was broken.

Review Video: Syntax
Visit mometrix.com/academy and enter code: 242280

Determining Meaning of Phrases and Paragraphs

Like unknown words, the meanings of phrases, paragraphs, and entire works can also be difficult to discern. Each of these can be better understood with added context. However, for larger groups of words, more context is needed. Unclear phrases are similar to unclear words, and the same methods can be used to understand their meaning. However, it is also important to consider how the individual words in the phrase work together. Paragraphs are a bit more complicated. Just as words must be compared to other words in a sentence, paragraphs must be compared to other paragraphs in a composition or a section.

Determining Meaning in Various Types of Compositions

To understand the meaning of an entire composition, the type of composition must be considered. **Expository writing** is generally organized so that each paragraph focuses on explaining one idea, or part of an idea, and its relevance. **Persuasive writing** uses paragraphs for different purposes to organize the parts of the argument. **Unclear paragraphs** must be read in the context of the paragraphs around them for their meaning to be fully understood. The meaning of full texts can also be unclear at times. The purpose of composition is also important for understanding the meaning of a text. To quickly understand the broad meaning of a text, look to the introductory and concluding paragraphs. Fictional texts are different. Some fictional works have implicit meanings, but some do not. The target audience must be considered for understanding texts that do have an implicit meaning, as most children's fiction will clearly state any lessons or morals. For other fiction, the application of literary theories and criticism may be helpful for understanding the text.

Resources for Determining Word Meaning and Usage

While these strategies are useful for determining the meaning of unknown words and phrases, sometimes additional resources are needed to properly use the terms in different contexts. Some words have multiple definitions, and some words are inappropriate in particular contexts or modes of writing. The following tools are helpful for understanding all meanings and proper uses for words and phrases.

- **Dictionaries** provide the meaning of a multitude of words in a language. Many dictionaries include additional information about each word, such as its etymology, its synonyms, or variations of the word.
- **Glossaries** are similar to dictionaries, as they provide the meanings of a variety of terms. However, while dictionaries typically feature an extensive list of words and comprise an entire publication, glossaries are often included at the end of a text and only include terms and definitions that are relevant to the text they follow.
- **Spell Checkers** are used to detect spelling errors in typed text. Some spell checkers may also detect the misuse of plural or singular nouns, verb tenses, or capitalization. While spell checkers are a helpful tool, they are not always reliable or attuned to the author's intent, so it is important to review the spell checker's suggestions before accepting them.
- **Style Manuals** are guidelines on the preferred punctuation, format, and grammar usage according to different fields or organizations. For example, the Associated Press Stylebook is a style guide often used for media writing. The guidelines within a style guide are not always applicable across different contexts and usages, as the guidelines often cover grammatical or formatting situations that are not objectively correct or incorrect.

Chapter Quiz

Ready to see how well you retained what you just read? Scan the QR code to go directly to the chapter quiz interface for this study guide. If you're using a computer, simply visit the bonus page at **mometrix.com/bonus948/kaplannursing** and click the Chapter Quizzes link.

Writing

Transform passive reading into active learning! After immersing yourself in this chapter, put your comprehension to the test by taking a quiz. The insights you gained will stay with you longer this way. Scan the QR code to go directly to the chapter quiz interface for this study guide. If you're using a computer, simply visit the bonus page at **mometrix.com/bonus948/kaplannursing** and click the Chapter Quizzes link.

The Writing Process

Brainstorming

Brainstorming is a technique that is used to find a creative approach to a subject. This can be accomplished by simple **free-association** with a topic. For example, with paper and pen, write every thought that you have about the topic in a word or phrase. This is done without critical thinking. You should put everything that comes to your mind about the topic on your scratch paper. Then, you need to read the list over a few times. Next, look for patterns, repetitions, and clusters of ideas. This allows a variety of fresh ideas to come as you think about the topic.

Free Writing

Free writing is a more structured form of brainstorming. The method involves taking a limited amount of time (e.g., 2 to 3 minutes) to write everything that comes to mind about the topic in complete sentences. When time expires, review everything that has been written down. Many of your sentences may make little or no sense, but the insights and observations that can come from free writing make this method a valuable approach. Usually, free writing results in a fuller expression of ideas than brainstorming because thoughts and associations are written in complete sentences. However, both techniques can be used to complement each other.

Planning

Planning is the process of organizing a piece of writing before composing a draft. Planning can include creating an outline or a graphic organizer, such as a Venn diagram, a spider-map, or a flowchart. These methods should help the writer identify their topic, main ideas, and the general organization of the composition. Preliminary research can also take place during this stage. Planning helps writers organize all of their ideas and decide if they have enough material to begin their first draft. However, writers should remember that the decisions they make during this step will likely change later in the process, so their plan does not have to be perfect.

Drafting

Writers may then use their plan, outline, or graphic organizer to compose their first draft. They may write subsequent drafts to improve their writing. Writing multiple drafts can help writers consider different ways to communicate their ideas and address errors that may be difficult to correct without rewriting a section or the whole composition. Most writers will vary in how many drafts they choose to write, as there is no "right" number of drafts. Writing drafts also takes away the pressure to write perfectly on the first try, as writers can improve with each draft they write.

Revising, Editing, and Proofreading

Once a writer completes a draft, they can move on to the revising, editing, and proofreading steps to improve their draft. These steps begin with making broad changes that may apply to large sections of a composition and then making small, specific corrections. **Revising** is the first and broadest of these steps. Revising involves ensuring that the composition addresses an appropriate audience, includes all necessary material, maintains focus throughout, and is organized logically. Revising may occur after the first draft to ensure that the following drafts improve upon errors from the first draft. Some revision should occur between each draft to avoid repeating these errors. The **editing** phase of writing is narrower than the revising phase. Editing a composition should include steps such as improving transitions between paragraphs, ensuring each paragraph is on topic, and improving the flow of the text. The editing phase may also include correcting grammatical errors that cannot be fixed without significantly altering the text. **Proofreading** involves fixing misspelled words, typos, other grammatical errors, and any remaining surface-level flaws in the composition.

Recursive Writing Process

However you approach writing, you may find comfort in knowing that the revision process can occur in any order. The **recursive writing process** is not as difficult as the phrase may make it seem. Simply put, the recursive writing process means that you may need to revisit steps after completing other steps. It also implies that the steps are not required to take place in any certain order. Indeed, you may find that planning, drafting, and revising can all take place at about the same time. The writing process involves moving back and forth between planning, drafting, and revising, followed by more planning, more drafting, and more revising until the writing is satisfactory.

Review Video: Recursive Writing Process
Visit mometrix.com/academy and enter code: 951611

Outlining and Organizing Ideas

Essays

Essays usually focus on one topic, subject, or goal. There are several types of essays, including informative, persuasive, and narrative. An essay's structure and level of formality depend on the type of essay and its goal. While narrative essays typically do not include outside sources, other types of essays often require some research and the integration of primary and secondary sources.

The basic format of an essay typically has three major parts: the introduction, the body, and the conclusion. The body is further divided into the writer's main points. Short and simple essays may have three main points, while essays covering broader ranges and going into more depth can have almost any number of main points, depending on length.

An essay's introduction should answer three questions:

1. What is the **subject** of the essay?

   If a student writes an essay about a book, the answer would include the title and author of the book and any additional information needed—such as the subject or argument of the book.

2. How does the essay **address** the subject?

To answer this, the writer identifies the essay's organization by briefly summarizing main points and the evidence supporting them.

3. What will the essay **prove**?

   This is the thesis statement, usually the opening paragraph's last sentence, clearly stating the writer's message.

The body elaborates on all the main points related to the thesis, introducing one main point at a time, and includes supporting evidence with each main point. Each body paragraph should state the point in a topic sentence, which is usually the first sentence in the paragraph. The paragraph should then explain the point's meaning, support it with quotations or other evidence, and then explain how this point and the evidence are related to the thesis. The writer should then repeat this procedure in a new paragraph for each additional main point.

The conclusion reiterates the content of the introduction, including the thesis, to remind the reader of the essay's main argument or subject. The essay writer may also summarize the highlights of the argument or description contained in the body of the essay, following the same sequence originally used in the body. For example, a conclusion might look like: Point 1 + Point 2 + Point 3 = Thesis, or Point 1 → Point 2 → Point 3 → Thesis Proof. Good organization makes essays easier for writers to compose and provides a guide for readers to follow. Well-organized essays hold attention better and are more likely to get readers to accept their theses as valid.

Main Ideas, Supporting Details, and Outlining a Topic

A writer often begins the first paragraph of a paper by stating the **main idea** or point, also known as the **topic sentence**. The rest of the paragraph supplies particular details that develop and support the main point. One way to visualize the relationship between the main point and supporting information is by considering a table: the tabletop is the main point, and each of the table's legs is a supporting detail or group of details. Both professional authors and students can benefit from planning their writing by first making an outline of the topic. Outlines facilitate quick identification of the main point and supporting details without having to wade through the additional language that will exist in the fully developed essay, article, or paper. Outlining can also help readers to analyze a piece of existing writing for the same reason. The outline first summarizes the main idea in one sentence. Then, below that, it summarizes the supporting details in a numbered list. Writing the paper then consists of filling in the outline with detail, writing a paragraph for each supporting point, and adding an introduction and conclusion.

Introduction

The purpose of the introduction is to capture the reader's attention and announce the essay's main idea. Normally, the introduction contains 50-80 words, or 3-5 sentences. An introduction can begin with an interesting quote, a question, or a strong opinion—something that will **engage** the reader's interest and prompt them to keep reading. If you are writing your essay to a specific prompt, your introduction should include a **restatement or summarization** of the prompt so that the reader will have some context for your essay. Finally, your introduction should briefly state your **thesis or main idea**: the primary thing you hope to communicate to the reader through your essay. Don't try to include all of the details and nuances of your thesis, or all of your reasons for it, in the introduction. That's what the rest of the essay is for!

Review Video: Introduction
Visit mometrix.com/academy and enter code: 961328

Thesis Statement

The thesis is the main idea of the essay. A temporary thesis, or working thesis, should be established early in the writing process because it will serve to keep the writer focused as ideas develop. This temporary thesis is subject to change as you continue to write.

The temporary thesis has two parts: a **topic** (i.e., the focus of your essay based on the prompt) and a **comment**. The comment makes an important point about the topic. A temporary thesis should be interesting and specific. Also, you need to limit the topic to a manageable scope. These three questions are useful tools to measure the effectiveness of any temporary thesis:

- Does the focus of my essay have enough interest to hold an audience?
- Is the focus of my essay specific enough to generate interest?
- Is the focus of my essay manageable for the time limit? Too broad? Too narrow?

The thesis should be a generalization rather than a fact because the thesis prepares readers for facts and details that support the thesis. The process of bringing the thesis into sharp focus may help in outlining major sections of the work. Once the thesis and introduction are complete, you can address the body of the work.

Review Video: Thesis Statements
Visit mometrix.com/academy and enter code: 691033

Supporting the Thesis

Throughout your essay, the thesis should be **explained clearly and supported** adequately by additional arguments. The thesis sentence needs to contain a clear statement of the purpose of your essay and a comment about the thesis. With the thesis statement, you have an opportunity to state what is noteworthy of this particular treatment of the prompt. Each sentence and paragraph should build on and support the thesis.

When you respond to the prompt, use parts of the passage to support your argument or defend your position. Using supporting evidence from the passage strengths your argument because readers can see your attention to the entire passage and your response to the details and facts within the passage. You can use facts, details, statistics, and direct quotations from the passage to uphold your position. Be sure to point out which information comes from the original passage and base your argument around that evidence.

Body

In an essay's introduction, the writer establishes the thesis and may indicate how the rest of the piece will be structured. In the body of the piece, the writer **elaborates** upon, **illustrates**, and **explains** the **thesis statement**. How writers arrange supporting details and their choices of paragraph types are development techniques. Writers may give examples of the concept introduced in the thesis statement. If the subject includes a cause-and-effect relationship, the author may explain its causality. A writer will explain or analyze the main idea of the piece throughout the body, often by presenting arguments for the veracity or credibility of the thesis statement. Writers may use development to define or clarify ambiguous terms. Paragraphs within the body may be organized using natural sequences, like space and time. Writers may employ **inductive reasoning**, using multiple details to establish a generalization or causal relationship, or **deductive reasoning**, proving a generalized hypothesis or proposition through a specific example or case.

Review Video: Drafting Body Paragraphs
Visit mometrix.com/academy and enter code: 724590

PARAGRAPHS

After the introduction of a passage, a series of body paragraphs will carry a message through to the conclusion. Each paragraph should be **unified around a main point**. Normally, a good topic sentence summarizes the paragraph's main point. A topic sentence is a general sentence that gives an introduction to the paragraph.

The sentences that follow support the topic sentence. However, though it is usually the first sentence, the topic sentence can come as the final sentence to the paragraph if the earlier sentences give a clear explanation of the paragraph's topic. This allows the topic sentence to function as a concluding sentence. Overall, the paragraphs need to stay true to the main point. This means that any unnecessary sentences that do not advance the main point should be removed.

The main point of a paragraph requires adequate development (i.e., a substantial paragraph that covers the main point). A paragraph of two or three sentences does not cover a main point. This is especially true when the main point of the paragraph gives strong support to the argument of the thesis. An occasional short paragraph is fine as a transitional device. However, a well-developed argument will have paragraphs with more than a few sentences.

METHODS OF DEVELOPING PARAGRAPHS

Common methods of adding substance to paragraphs include examples, illustrations, analogies, and cause and effect.

- **Examples** are supporting details to the main idea of a paragraph or a passage. When authors write about something that their audience may not understand, they can provide an example to show their point. When authors write about something that is not easily accepted, they can give examples to prove their point.
- **Illustrations** are extended examples that require several sentences. Well-selected illustrations can be a great way for authors to develop a point that may not be familiar to their audience.
- **Analogies** make comparisons between items that appear to have nothing in common. Analogies are employed by writers to provoke fresh thoughts about a subject. These comparisons may be used to explain the unfamiliar, to clarify an abstract point, or to argue a point. Although analogies are effective literary devices, they should be used carefully in arguments. Two things may be alike in some respects but completely different in others.
- **Cause and effect** is an excellent device to explain the connection between an action or situation and a particular result. One way that authors can use cause and effect is to state the effect in the topic sentence of a paragraph and add the causes in the body of the paragraph. This method can give an author's paragraphs structure, which always strengthens writing.

TYPES OF PARAGRAPHS

- A **paragraph of narration** tells a story or a part of a story. Normally, the sentences are arranged in chronological order (i.e., the order that the events happened). However, flashbacks (i.e., an anecdote from an earlier time) can be included.

- A **descriptive paragraph** makes a verbal portrait of a person, place, or thing. When specific details are used that appeal to one or more of the senses (i.e., sight, sound, smell, taste, and touch), authors give readers a sense of being present in the moment.
- A **process paragraph** is related to time order (i.e., First, you open the bottle. Second, you pour the liquid, etc.). Usually, this describes a process or teaches readers how to perform a process.
- **Comparing two things** draws attention to their similarities and indicates a number of differences. When authors contrast, they focus only on differences. Both comparing and contrasting may be done point-by-point, noting both the similarities and differences of each point, or in sequential paragraphs, where you discuss all the similarities and then all the differences, or vice versa.

Breaking Text into Paragraphs

For most forms of writing, you will need to use multiple paragraphs. As such, determining when to start a new paragraph is very important. Reasons for starting a new paragraph include:

- To mark off the introduction and concluding paragraphs
- To signal a shift to a new idea or topic
- To indicate an important shift in time or place
- To explain a point in additional detail
- To highlight a comparison, contrast, or cause and effect relationship

Paragraph Length

Most readers find that their comfort level for a paragraph is between 100 and 200 words. Shorter paragraphs cause too much starting and stopping and give a choppy effect. Paragraphs that are too long often test the attention span of readers. Two notable exceptions to this rule exist. In scientific or scholarly papers, longer paragraphs suggest seriousness and depth. In journalistic writing, constraints are placed on paragraph size by the narrow columns in a newspaper format.

The first and last paragraphs of a text will usually be the introduction and conclusion. These special-purpose paragraphs are likely to be shorter than paragraphs in the body of the work. Paragraphs in the body of the essay follow the subject's outline (e.g., one paragraph per point in short essays and a group of paragraphs per point in longer works). Some ideas require more development than others, so it is good for a writer to remain flexible. A paragraph of excessive length may be divided, and shorter ones may be combined.

Conclusion

Two important principles to consider when writing a conclusion are strength and closure. A strong conclusion gives the reader a sense that the author's main points are meaningful and important, and that the supporting facts and arguments are convincing, solid, and well developed. When a conclusion achieves closure, it gives the impression that the writer has stated all necessary information and points and completed the work, rather than simply stopping after a specified length. Some things to avoid when writing concluding paragraphs include:

- Introducing a completely new idea
- Beginning with obvious or unoriginal phrases like "In conclusion" or "To summarize"
- Apologizing for one's opinions or writing
- Repeating the thesis word for word rather than rephrasing it
- Believing that the conclusion must always summarize the piece

Coherence in Writing

Coherent Paragraphs

A smooth flow of sentences and paragraphs without gaps, shifts, or bumps will lead to paragraph **coherence**. Ties between old and new information can be smoothed using several methods:

- **Linking ideas clearly**, from the topic sentence to the body of the paragraph, is essential for a smooth transition. The topic sentence states the main point, and this should be followed by specific details, examples, and illustrations that support the topic sentence. The support may be direct or indirect. In **indirect support**, the illustrations and examples may support a sentence that in turn supports the topic directly.
- The **repetition of key words** adds coherence to a paragraph. To avoid dull language, variations of the key words may be used.
- **Parallel structures** are often used within sentences to emphasize the similarity of ideas and connect sentences giving similar information.
- Maintaining a **consistent verb tense** throughout the paragraph helps. Shifting tenses affects the smooth flow of words and can disrupt the coherence of the paragraph.

Review Video: How to Write a Good Paragraph
Visit mometrix.com/academy and enter code: 682127

Sequence Words and Phrases

When a paragraph opens with the topic sentence, the second sentence may begin with a phrase like *first of all*, introducing the first supporting detail or example. The writer may introduce the second supporting item with words or phrases like *also, in addition*, and *besides*. The writer might introduce succeeding pieces of support with wording like, *another thing, moreover, furthermore*, or *not only that, but*. The writer may introduce the last piece of support with *lastly, finally*, or *last but not least*. Writers get off the point by presenting off-target items not supporting the main point. For example, a main point *my dog is not smart* is supported by the statement, *he's six years old and still doesn't answer to his name*. But *he cries when I leave for school* is not supportive, as it does not indicate lack of intelligence. Writers stay on point by presenting only supportive statements that are directly relevant to and illustrative of their main point.

Review Video: Sequence
Visit mometrix.com/academy and enter code: 489027

Transitions

Transitions between sentences and paragraphs guide readers from idea to idea and indicate relationships between sentences and paragraphs. Writers should be judicious in their use of transitions, inserting them sparingly. They should also be selected to fit the author's purpose—transitions can indicate time, comparison, and conclusion, among other purposes. Tone is also important to consider when using transitional phrases, varying the tone for different audiences. For example, in a scholarly essay, *in summary* would be preferable to the more informal *in short*.

When working with transitional words and phrases, writers usually find a natural flow that indicates when a transition is needed. In reading a draft of the text, it should become apparent where the flow is disrupted. At this point, the writer can add transitional elements during the revision process. Revising can also afford an opportunity to delete transitional devices that seem heavy handed or unnecessary.

Review Video: Transitions in Writing
Visit mometrix.com/academy and enter code: 233246

TYPES OF TRANSITIONAL WORDS

Time	afterward, immediately, earlier, meanwhile, recently, lately, now, since, soon, when, then, until, before, etc.
Sequence	too, first, second, further, moreover, also, again, and, next, still, besides, finally
Comparison	similarly, in the same way, likewise, also, again, once more
Contrasting	but, although, despite, however, instead, nevertheless, on the one hand... on the other hand, regardless, yet, in contrast
Cause and Effect	because, consequently, thus, therefore, then, to this end, since, so, as a result, if... then, accordingly
Examples	for example, for instance, such as, to illustrate, indeed, in fact, specifically
Place	near, far, here, there, to the left/right, next to, above, below, beyond, opposite, beside
Concession	granted that, naturally, of course, it may appear, although it is true that
Repetition, Summary, or Conclusion	as mentioned earlier, as noted, in other words, in short, on the whole, to summarize, therefore, as a result, to conclude, in conclusion
Addition	and, also, furthermore, moreover
Generalization	in broad terms, broadly speaking, in general

Review Video: Transition Words
Visit mometrix.com/academy and enter code: 707563

Review Video: How to Effectively Connect Sentences
Visit mometrix.com/academy and enter code: 948325

Writing Style and Form

WRITING STYLE AND LINGUISTIC FORM

Linguistic form encodes the literal meanings of words and sentences. It comes from the phonological, morphological, syntactic, and semantic parts of a language. **Writing style** consists of different ways of encoding the meaning and indicating figurative and stylistic meanings. An author's writing style can also be referred to as his or her **voice**.

Writers' stylistic choices accomplish three basic effects on their audiences:

- They **communicate meanings** beyond linguistically dictated meanings,
- They communicate the **author's attitude**, such as persuasive or argumentative effects accomplished through style, and
- They communicate or **express feelings**.

Within style, component areas include:

- Narrative structure
- Viewpoint
- Focus

- Sound patterns
- Meter and rhythm
- Lexical and syntactic repetition and parallelism
- Writing genre
- Representational, realistic, and mimetic effects
- Representation of thought and speech
- Meta-representation (representing representation)
- Irony
- Metaphor and other indirect meanings
- Representation and use of historical and dialectal variations
- Gender-specific and other group-specific speech styles, both real and fictitious
- Analysis of the processes for inferring meaning from writing

TONE

Tone may be defined as the writer's **attitude** toward the topic, and to the audience. This attitude is reflected in the language used in the writing. The tone of a work should be **appropriate to the topic** and to the intended audience. While it may be fine to use slang or jargon in some pieces, other texts should not contain such terms. Tone can range from humorous to serious and any level in between. It may be more or less formal, depending on the purpose of the writing and its intended audience. All these nuances in tone can flavor the entire writing and should be kept in mind as the work evolves.

Review Video: Style, Tone, and Mood
Visit mometrix.com/academy and enter code: 416961

WORD SELECTION

A writer's choice of words is a signature of their style. Careful thought about the use of words can improve a piece of writing. A passage can be an exciting piece to read when attention is given to the use of vivid or specific nouns rather than general ones.

Example:

General: His kindness will never be forgotten.

Specific: His thoughtful gifts and bear hugs will never be forgotten.

ACTIVE AND PASSIVE LANGUAGE

Attention should also be given to the kind of verbs that are used in sentences. Active verbs (e.g., run, swim) are about an action. Whenever possible, an **active verb should replace a linking verb** to provide clear examples for arguments and to strengthen a passage overall. When using an active verb, one should be sure that the verb is used in the active voice instead of the passive voice. Verbs are in the active voice when the subject is the one doing the action. A verb is in the passive voice when the subject is the recipient of an action.

Example:

Passive: The winners were called to the stage by the judges.

Active: The judges called the winners to the stage.

Conciseness

Conciseness is writing that communicates a message in the fewest words possible. Writing concisely is valuable because short, uncluttered messages allow the reader to understand the author's message more easily and efficiently. Planning is important in writing concise messages. If you have in mind what you need to write beforehand, it will be easier to make a message short and to the point. Do not state the obvious.

Revising is also important. After the message is written, make sure you have effective, pithy sentences that efficiently get your point across. When reviewing the information, imagine a conversation taking place, and concise writing will likely result.

Appropriate Kinds of Writing for Different Tasks, Purposes, and Audiences

When preparing to write a composition, consider the audience and purpose to choose the best type of writing. Four common types of writing are persuasive, expository, and narrative. **Persuasive**, or argumentative writing, is used to convince the audience to take action or agree with the author's claims. **Expository** writing is meant to inform the audience of the author's observations or research on a topic. **Narrative** writing is used to tell the audience a story and often allows more room for creativity. **Descriptive** writing is when a writer provides a substantial amount of detail to the reader so he or she can visualize the topic. While task, purpose, and audience inform a writer's mode of writing, these factors also impact elements such as tone, vocabulary, and formality.

For example, students who are writing to persuade their parents to grant them some additional privilege, such as permission for a more independent activity, should use more sophisticated vocabulary and diction that sounds more mature and serious to appeal to the parental audience. However, students who are writing for younger children should use simpler vocabulary and sentence structure, as well as choose words that are more vivid and entertaining. They should treat their topics more lightly, and include humor when appropriate. Students who are writing for their classmates may use language that is more informal, as well as age-appropriate.

Review Video: Writing Purpose and Audience
Visit mometrix.com/academy and enter code: 146627

Formality in Writing

Level of Formality

The relationship between writer and reader is important in choosing a **level of formality** as most writing requires some degree of formality. **Formal writing** is for addressing a superior in a school or work environment. Business letters, textbooks, and newspapers use a moderate to high level of formality. **Informal writing** is appropriate for private letters, personal emails, and business correspondence between close associates.

For your exam, you will want to be aware of informal and formal writing. One way that this can be accomplished is to watch for shifts in point of view in the essay. For example, unless writers are using a personal example, they will rarely refer to themselves (e.g., "*I* think that *my* point is very clear.") to avoid being informal when they need to be formal.

Also, be mindful of an author who addresses his or her audience **directly** in their writing (e.g., "Readers, *like you*, will understand this argument.") as this can be a sign of informal writing. Good writers understand the need to be consistent with their level of formality. Shifts in levels of formality or point of view can confuse readers and cause them to discount the message.

CLICHÉS

Clichés are phrases that have been **overused** to the point that the phrase has no importance or has lost the original meaning. These phrases have no originality and add very little to a passage. Therefore, most writers will avoid the use of clichés. Another option is to make changes to a cliché so that it is not predictable and empty of meaning.

Examples:

> When life gives you lemons, make lemonade.
>
> Every cloud has a silver lining.

JARGON

Jargon is **specialized vocabulary** that is used among members of a certain trade or profession. Since jargon is understood by only a small audience, writers will use jargon in passages that will only be read by a specialized audience. For example, medical jargon should be used in a medical journal but not in a New York Times article. Jargon includes exaggerated language that tries to impress rather than inform. Sentences filled with jargon are not precise and are difficult to understand.

Examples:

> "He is going to *toenail* these frames for us." (Toenail is construction jargon for nailing at an angle.)
>
> "They brought in a *kip* of material today." (Kip refers to 1000 pounds in architecture and engineering.)

SLANG

Slang is an **informal** and sometimes private language that is understood by some individuals. Slang terms have some usefulness, but they can have a small audience. So, most formal writing will not include this kind of language.

Examples:

> "Yes, the event was a blast!" (In this sentence, *blast* means that the event was a great experience.)
>
> "That attempt was an epic fail." (By *epic fail*, the speaker means that his or her attempt was not a success.)

COLLOQUIALISM

A colloquialism is a word or phrase that is found in informal writing. Unlike slang, **colloquial language** will be familiar to a greater range of people. However, colloquialisms are still considered inappropriate for formal writing. Colloquial language can include some slang, but these are limited to contractions for the most part.

Examples:

> "Can *y'all* come back another time?" (Y'all is a contraction of "you all.")
>
> "Will you stop him from building this *castle in the air*?" (A "castle in the air" is an improbable or unlikely event.)

ACADEMIC LANGUAGE

In educational settings, students are often expected to use academic language in their schoolwork. Academic language is also commonly found in dissertations and theses, texts published by academic journals, and other forms of academic research. Academic language conventions may vary between fields, but general academic language is free of slang, regional terminology, and noticeable grammatical errors. Specific terms may also be used in academic language, and it is important to understand their proper usage. A writer's command of academic language impacts their ability to communicate in an academic or professional context. While it is acceptable to use colloquialisms, slang, improper grammar, or other forms of informal speech in social settings or at home, it is inappropriate to practice non-academic language in academic contexts.

Common Types of Writing

AUTOBIOGRAPHICAL NARRATIVES

Autobiographical narratives are narratives written by an author about an event or period in their life. Autobiographical narratives are written from one person's perspective, in first person, and often include the author's thoughts and feelings alongside their description of the event or period. Structure, style, or theme varies between different autobiographical narratives, since each narrative is personal and specific to its author and his or her experience.

REFLECTIVE ESSAY

A less common type of essay is the reflective essay. **Reflective essays** allow the author to reflect, or think back, on an experience and analyze what they recall. They should consider what they learned from the experience, what they could have done differently, what would have helped them during the experience, or anything else that they have realized from looking back on the experience. Reflection essays incorporate both objective reflection on one's own actions and subjective explanation of thoughts and feelings. These essays can be written for a number of experiences in a formal or informal context.

JOURNALS AND DIARIES

A **journal** is a personal account of events, experiences, feelings, and thoughts. Many people write journals to express their feelings and thoughts or to help them process experiences they have had. Since journals are **private documents** not meant to be shared with others, writers may not be concerned with grammar, spelling, or other mechanics. However, authors may write journals that they expect or hope to publish someday; in this case, they not only express their thoughts and feelings and process their experiences, but they also attend to their craft in writing them. Some authors compose journals to record a particular time period or a series of related events, such as a cancer diagnosis, treatment, surviving the disease, and how these experiences have changed or affected them. Other experiences someone might include in a journal are recovering from addiction, journeys of spiritual exploration and discovery, time spent in another country, or anything else someone wants to personally document. Journaling can also be therapeutic, as some people use journals to work through feelings of grief over loss or to wrestle with big decisions.

EXAMPLES OF DIARIES IN LITERATURE

The Diary of a Young Girl by Dutch Jew Anne Frank (1947) contains her life-affirming, nonfictional diary entries from 1942-1944 while her family hid in an attic from World War II's genocidal Nazis. *Go Ask Alice* (1971) by Beatrice Sparks is a cautionary, fictional novel in the form of diary entries by Alice, an unhappy, rebellious teen who takes LSD, runs away from home and lives with hippies, and eventually returns home. Frank's writing reveals an intelligent, sensitive, insightful girl, raised by intellectual European parents—a girl who believes in the goodness of human nature despite surrounding atrocities. Alice, influenced by early 1970s counterculture, becomes less optimistic. However, similarities can be found between them: Frank dies in a Nazi concentration camp while the fictitious Alice dies from a drug overdose. Both young women are also unable to escape their surroundings. Additionally, adolescent searches for personal identity are evident in both books.

Review Video: Journals, Diaries, Letters, and Blogs
Visit mometrix.com/academy and enter code: 432845

LETTERS

Letters are messages written to other people. In addition to letters written between individuals, some writers compose letters to the editors of newspapers, magazines, and other publications, while some write "Open Letters" to be published and read by the general public. Open letters, while intended for everyone to read, may also identify a group of people or a single person whom the letter directly addresses. In everyday use, the most-used forms are business letters and personal or friendly letters. Both kinds share common elements: business or personal letterhead stationery; the writer's return address at the top; the addressee's address next; a salutation, such as "Dear [name]" or some similar opening greeting, followed by a colon in business letters or a comma in personal letters; the body of the letter, with paragraphs as indicated; and a closing, like "Sincerely/Cordially/Best regards/etc." or "Love," in intimate personal letters.

EARLY LETTERS

The Greek word for "letter" is *epistolē*, which became the English word "epistle." The earliest letters were called epistles, including the New Testament's epistles from the apostles to the Christians. In ancient Egypt, the writing curriculum in scribal schools included the epistolary genre. Epistolary novels frame a story in the form of letters. Examples of noteworthy epistolary novels include:

- *Pamela* (1740), by 18th-century English novelist Samuel Richardson
- *Shamela* (1741), Henry Fielding's satire of *Pamela* that mocked epistolary writing.
- *Lettres persanes* (1721) by French author Montesquieu
- *The Sorrows of Young Werther* (1774) by German author Johann Wolfgang von Goethe
- *The History of Emily Montague* (1769), the first Canadian novel, by Frances Brooke
- *Dracula* (1897) by Bram Stoker
- *Frankenstein* (1818) by Mary Shelley
- *The Color Purple* (1982) by Alice Walker

BLOGS

The word "blog" is derived from "weblog" and refers to writing done exclusively on the internet. Readers of reputable newspapers expect quality content and layouts that enable easy reading. These expectations also apply to blogs. For example, readers can easily move visually from line to line when columns are narrow, while overly wide columns cause readers to lose their places. Blogs must also be posted with layouts enabling online readers to follow them easily. However, because the way people read on computer, tablet, and smartphone screens differs from how they read print on paper, formatting and writing blog content is more complex than writing newspaper articles. Two major principles are the bases for blog-writing rules: The first is while readers of print articles skim to estimate their length, online they must scroll down to scan; therefore, blog layouts need more subheadings, graphics, and other indications of what information follows. The second is onscreen reading can be harder on the eyes than reading printed paper, so legibility is crucial in blogs.

Rules and Rationales for Writing Blogs

1. Format all posts for smooth page layout and easy scanning.
2. Column width should not be too wide, as larger lines of text can be difficult to read
3. Headings and subheadings separate text visually, enable scanning or skimming, and encourage continued reading.
4. Bullet-pointed or numbered lists enable quick information location and scanning.
5. Punctuation is critical, so beginners should use shorter sentences until confident in their knowledge of punctuation rules.
6. Blog paragraphs should be far shorter—two to six sentences each—than paragraphs written on paper to enable "chunking" because reading onscreen is more difficult.
7. Sans-serif fonts are usually clearer than serif fonts, and larger font sizes are better.
8. Highlight important material and draw attention with **boldface**, but avoid overuse. Avoid hard-to-read *italics* and ALL CAPITALS.
9. Include enough blank spaces: overly busy blogs tire eyes and brains. Images not only break up text but also emphasize and enhance text and can attract initial reader attention.
10. Use background colors judiciously to avoid distracting the eye or making it difficult to read.
11. Be consistent throughout posts, since people read them in different orders.
12. Tell a story with a beginning, middle, and end.

Specialized Types of Writing

Editorials

Editorials are articles in newspapers, magazines, and other serial publications. Editorials express an opinion or belief belonging to the majority of the publication's leadership. This opinion or belief generally refers to a specific issue, topic, or event. These articles are authored by a member, or a small number of members, of the publication's leadership and are often written to affect their readers, such as persuading them to adopt a stance or take a particular action.

Resumes

Resumes are brief, but formal, documents that outline an individual's experience in a certain area. Resumes are most often used for job applications. Such resumes will list the applicant's work experience, certification, and achievements or qualifications related to the position. Resumes should only include the most pertinent information. They should also use strategic formatting to highlight the applicant's most impressive experiences and achievements, to ensure the document can be read quickly and easily, and to eliminate both visual clutter and excessive negative space.

Reports

Reports summarize the results of research, new methodology, or other developments in an academic or professional context. Reports often include details about methodology and outside influences and factors. However, a report should focus primarily on the results of the research or development. Reports are objective and deliver information efficiently, sacrificing style for clear and effective communication.

MEMORANDA

A memorandum, also called a memo, is a formal method of communication used in professional settings. Memoranda are printed documents that include a heading listing the sender and their job title, the recipient and their job title, the date, and a specific subject line. Memoranda often include an introductory section explaining the reason and context for the memorandum. Next, a memorandum includes a section with details relevant to the topic. Finally, the memorandum will conclude with a paragraph that politely and clearly defines the sender's expectations of the recipient.

Technology in the Writing Process

Modern technology has yielded several tools that can be used to make the writing process more convenient and organized. Word processors and online tools, such as databases and plagiarism detectors, allow much of the writing process to be completed in one place, using one device.

TECHNOLOGY FOR PLANNING AND DRAFTING

For the planning and drafting stages of the writing process, word processors are a helpful tool. These programs also feature formatting tools, allowing users to create their own planning tools or create digital outlines that can be easily converted into sentences, paragraphs, or an entire essay draft. Online databases and references also complement the planning process by providing convenient access to information and sources for research. Word processors also allow users to keep up with their work and update it more easily than if they wrote their work by hand. Online word processors often allow users to collaborate, making group assignments more convenient. These programs also allow users to include illustrations or other supplemental media in their compositions.

TECHNOLOGY FOR REVISING, EDITING, AND PROOFREADING

Word processors also benefit the revising, editing, and proofreading stages of the writing process. Most of these programs indicate errors in spelling and grammar, allowing users to catch minor errors and correct them quickly. There are also websites designed to help writers by analyzing text for deeper errors, such as poor sentence structure, inappropriate complexity, lack of sentence variety, and style issues. These websites can help users fix errors they may not know to look for or may have simply missed. As writers finish these steps, they may benefit from checking their work for any plagiarism. There are several websites and programs that compare text to other documents and publications across the internet and detect any similarities within the text. These websites show the source of the similar information, so users know whether or not they referenced the source and unintentionally plagiarized its contents.

TECHNOLOGY FOR PUBLISHING

Technology also makes managing written work more convenient. Digitally storing documents keeps everything in one place and is easy to reference. Digital storage also makes sharing work easier, as documents can be attached to an email or stored online. This also allows writers to publish their work easily, as they can electronically submit it to other publications or freely post it to a personal blog, profile, or website.

Chapter Quiz

Ready to see how well you retained what you just read? Scan the QR code to go directly to the chapter quiz interface for this study guide. If you're using a computer, simply visit the bonus page at **mometrix.com/bonus948/kaplannursing** and click the Chapter Quizzes link.

Mathematics

Fundamental Math Skills

Number Basics

Classifications of Numbers

Numbers are the basic building blocks of mathematics. Specific features of numbers are identified by the following terms:

Integer – any positive or negative whole number, including zero. Integers do not include fractions $\left(\frac{1}{3}\right)$, decimals (0.56), or mixed numbers $\left(7\frac{3}{4}\right)$.

Prime number – any whole number greater than 1 that has only two factors, itself and 1; that is, a number that can be divided evenly only by 1 and itself.

Composite number – any whole number greater than 1 that has more than two different factors; in other words, any whole number that is not a prime number. For example: The composite number 8 has the factors of 1, 2, 4, and 8.

Even number – any integer that can be divided by 2 without leaving a remainder. For example: 2, 4, 6, 8, and so on.

Odd number – any integer that cannot be divided evenly by 2. For example: 3, 5, 7, 9, and so on.

Decimal number – any number that uses a decimal point to show the part of the number that is less than one. Example: 1.234.

Decimal point – a symbol used to separate the ones place from the tenths place in decimals or dollars from cents in currency.

Decimal place – the position of a number to the right of the decimal point. In the decimal 0.123, the 1 is in the first place to the right of the decimal point, indicating tenths; the 2 is in the second place, indicating hundredths; and the 3 is in the third place, indicating thousandths.

The **decimal**, or base 10, system is a number system that uses ten different digits (0, 1, 2, 3, 4, 5, 6, 7, 8, 9). An example of a number system that uses something other than ten digits is the **binary**, or base 2, number system, used by computers, which uses only the numbers 0 and 1. It is thought that the decimal system originated because people had only their 10 fingers for counting.

Rational numbers include all integers, decimals, and fractions. Any terminating or repeating decimal number is a rational number.

Irrational numbers cannot be written as fractions or decimals because the number of decimal places is infinite and there is no recurring pattern of digits within the number. For example, pi (π) begins with 3.141592 and continues without terminating or repeating, so pi is an irrational number.

Real numbers are the set of all rational and irrational numbers.

Review Video: Classification of Numbers
Visit mometrix.com/academy and enter code: 461071

Review Video: Prime and Composite Numbers
Visit mometrix.com/academy and enter code: 565581

Numbers in Word Form and Place Value

When writing numbers out in word form or translating word form to numbers, it is essential to understand how a place value system works. In the decimal or base-10 system, each digit of a number represents how many of the corresponding place value—a specific factor of 10—are contained in the number being represented. To make reading numbers easier, every three digits to the left of the decimal place is preceded by a comma. The following table demonstrates some of the place values:

Power of 10	10^3	10^2	10^1	10^0	10^{-1}	10^{-2}	10^{-3}
Value	1,000	100	10	1	0.1	0.01	0.001
Place	thousands	hundreds	tens	ones	tenths	hundredths	thousandths

For example, consider the number 4,546.09, which can be separated into each place value like this:

4: thousands
5: hundreds
4: tens
6: ones
0: tenths
9: hundredths

This number in word form would be *four thousand five hundred forty-six and nine hundredths.*

Review Video: Place Value
Visit mometrix.com/academy and enter code: 205433

Rounding and Estimation

Rounding is reducing the digits in a number while still trying to keep the value similar. The result will be less accurate but in a simpler form and easier to use. Whole numbers can be rounded to the nearest ten, hundred, or thousand, for instance.

To round a number, we make it a little smaller (rounding down) or a little larger (rounding up) to get a number that ends in zeros. We specify the number of zeros by naming the last place that we will not "zero out." For example, to round 8,3̲27 to the nearest hundred, we round down to 8,3̲00, zeroing out every digit to the right of the hundreds place. To round 4̲,728 to the nearest thousand, we round up to 5̲,000, increasing the thousands digit by one (to make the number larger) and zeroing out every digit to the right of the thousands place.

We decide whether to round down or up by looking at the first digit we are going to zero out. If it is less than 5 (namely, 0, 1, 2, 3, or 4) we round down. If it is greater than or equal to 5 (namely, 5, 6, 7, 8, or 9) we round up by adding 1 to the place we are rounding to. So, rounding 8,3̲27 to the nearest hundred, we round down to 8,3̲00 because the tens digit, 2, is less than 5. And rounding 4̲,728 to the nearest thousand, we round up to 5,000, increasing the thousands digit by 1, because the hundreds digit, 7, is greater than or equal to 5.

This even works with decimals. For example, rounding 39.7426 to the nearest tenth, we round down to 39.7000 (or simply 39.7) because the hundredths digit, 4, is less than 5. And rounding 0.019823 to the nearest thousandth, we round up to 0.020000 (or simply 0.02) by increasing the thousandths digit by 1, because the ten-thousandths digit, 8, is greater than or equal to 5.

When you are asked to estimate the solution to a problem, you will need to provide only an approximate figure or **estimation** for your answer. In this situation, you will need to round each number in the calculation to the level indicated (nearest hundred, nearest thousand, etc.) or to a level that makes sense for the numbers involved. When estimating a sum **all numbers must be rounded to the same level**. You cannot round one number to the nearest thousand while rounding another to the nearest hundred.

For instance, suppose you are considering buying four pieces of equipment for your home office. Their prices are $485, $1,217, $750, and $643. To estimate their total cost, you might round each price to the nearest hundred and add the rounded figures, getting an estimate of $500 + $1,200 + $800 + $600 = $3,100. By estimating instead of making an exact calculation, you give up a little accuracy to get a simpler calculation.

Review Video: Rounding and Estimation
Visit mometrix.com/academy and enter code: 126243

Absolute Value

A precursor to working with negative numbers is understanding what **absolute values** are. A number's absolute value is simply the distance away from zero a number is on the number line. The absolute value of a number is always positive and is written $|x|$. For example, the absolute value of 3, written as $|3|$, is 3 because the distance between 0 and 3 on a number line is three units. Likewise, the absolute value of -3, written as $|-3|$, is 3 because the distance between 0 and -3 on a number line is three units. So $|3| = |-3|$.

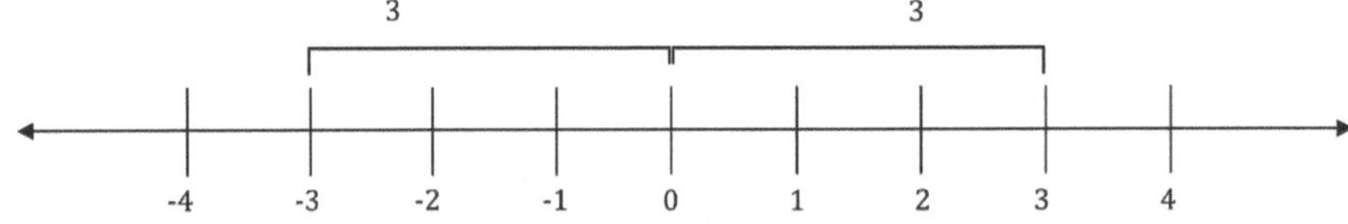

Review Video: Absolute Value
Visit mometrix.com/academy and enter code: 314669

Operations

An **operation** is simply a mathematical process that takes some value(s) as input(s) and produces an output. Elementary operations are often written in the following form: *value operation value*. For instance, in the expression $1 + 2$ the values are 1 and 2 and the operation is addition. Performing the operation gives the output of 3. In this way we can say that $1 + 2$ and 3 are equal, or $1 + 2 = 3$.

Addition

Addition increases the value of one quantity by the value of another quantity (both called **addends**). Example: $2 + 4 = 6$ or $8 + 9 = 17$. The result is called the **sum**. With addition, the order does not matter, $4 + 2 = 2 + 4$.

When adding signed numbers, if the signs are the same simply add the absolute values of the addends and apply the original sign to the sum. For example, $(+4) + (+8) = +12$ and $(-4) + (-8) = -12$. When the original signs are different, take the absolute values of the addends and subtract the smaller value from the larger value, then apply the original sign of the larger value to the difference. Example: $(+4) + (-8) = -4$ and $(-4) + (+8) = +4$.

Subtraction

Subtraction is the opposite operation to addition; it decreases the value of one quantity (the **minuend**) by the value of another quantity (the **subtrahend**). For example, $6 - 4 = 2$ or $17 - 8 = 9$. The result is called the **difference**. Note that with subtraction, the order does matter, $6 - 4 \neq 4 - 6$.

For subtracting signed numbers, change the sign of the subtrahend and then follow the same rules used for addition. Example: $(+4) - (+8) = (+4) + (-8) = -4$

Multiplication

Multiplication can be thought of as repeated addition. One number (the **multiplier**) indicates how many times to add the other number (the **multiplicand**) to itself. Example: $3 \times 2 = 2 + 2 + 2 = 6$. With multiplication, the order does not matter, $2 \times 3 = 3 \times 2$ or $3 + 3 = 2 + 2 + 2$, either way the result (the **product**) is the same.

If the signs are the same, the product is positive when multiplying signed numbers. Example: $(+4) \times (+8) = +32$ and $(-4) \times (-8) = +32$. If the signs are opposite, the product is negative. Example: $(+4) \times (-8) = -32$ and $(-4) \times (+8) = -32$. When more than two factors are multiplied together, the sign of the product is determined by how many negative factors are present. If there are an odd number of negative factors then the product is negative, whereas an even number of negative factors indicates a positive product. Example: $(+4) \times (-8) \times (-2) = +64$ and $(-4) \times (-8) \times (-2) = -64$.

Division

Division is the opposite operation to multiplication; one number (the **divisor**) tells us how many parts to divide the other number (the **dividend**) into. The result of division is called the **quotient**. Example: $20 \div 4 = 5$. If 20 is split into 4 equal parts, each part is 5. With division, the order of the numbers does matter, $20 \div 4 \neq 4 \div 20$.

The rules for dividing signed numbers are similar to multiplying signed numbers. If the dividend and divisor have the same sign, the quotient is positive. If the dividend and divisor have opposite signs, the quotient is negative. Example: $(-4) \div (+8) = -0.5$.

> **Review Video: Mathematical Operations**
> Visit mometrix.com/academy and enter code: 208095

Parentheses

Parentheses are used to designate which operations should be done first when there are multiple operations. Example: $4 - (2 + 1) = 1$; the parentheses tell us that we must add 2 and 1, and then subtract the sum from 4, rather than subtracting 2 from 4 and then adding 1 (this would give us an answer of 3).

> **Review Video: Mathematical Parentheses**
> Visit mometrix.com/academy and enter code: 978600

EXPONENTS

An **exponent** is a superscript number placed next to another number at the top right. It indicates how many times the base number is to be multiplied by itself. Exponents provide a shorthand way to write what would be a longer mathematical expression, Example: $2^4 = 2 \times 2 \times 2 \times 2$. A number with an exponent of 2 is said to be "squared," while a number with an exponent of 3 is said to be "cubed." The value of a number raised to an exponent is called its power. So 8^4 is read as "8 to the 4th power," or "8 raised to the power of 4."

> **Review Video: Exponents**
> Visit mometrix.com/academy and enter code: 600998

ROOTS

A **root**, such as a square root, is another way of writing a fractional exponent. Instead of using a superscript, roots use the radical symbol ($\sqrt{\ }$) to indicate the operation. A radical will have a number underneath the bar, and may sometimes have a number in the upper left: $\sqrt[n]{a}$, read as "the nth root of a." The relationship between radical notation and exponent notation can be described by this equation:

$$\sqrt[n]{a} = a^{\frac{1}{n}}$$

The two special cases of $n = 2$ and $n = 3$ are called square roots and cube roots. If there is no number to the upper left, the radical is understood to be a square root ($n = 2$). Nearly all of the roots you encounter will be square roots. A square root is the same as a number raised to the one-half power. When we say that a is the square root of b ($a = \sqrt{b}$), we mean that a multiplied by itself equals b: ($a \times a = b$).

A **perfect square** is a number that has an integer for its square root. There are 10 perfect squares from 1 to 100: 1, 4, 9, 16, 25, 36, 49, 64, 81, 100 (the squares of integers 1 through 10).

> **Review Video: Roots**
> Visit mometrix.com/academy and enter code: 795655
>
> **Review Video: Perfect Squares and Square Roots**
> Visit mometrix.com/academy and enter code: 648063

WORD PROBLEMS AND MATHEMATICAL SYMBOLS

When working on word problems, you must be able to translate verbal expressions or "math words" into math symbols. This chart contains several "math words" and their appropriate symbols:

Phrase	Symbol
equal, is, was, will be, has, costs, gets to, is the same as, becomes	$=$
times, of, multiplied by, product of, twice, doubles, halves, triples	$\times$
divided by, per, ratio of/to, out of	$\div$
plus, added to, sum, combined, and, more than, totals of	$+$
subtracted from, less than, decreased by, minus, difference between	$-$
what, how much, original value, how many, a number, a variable	x, n, etc.

Review Video: Understanding Word Problems
Visit mometrix.com/academy and enter code: 499199

Examples of Translated Mathematical Phrases

- The phrase four more than twice a number can be written algebraically as $2x + 4$.
- The phrase half a number decreased by six can be written algebraically as $\frac{1}{2}x - 6$.
- The phrase the sum of a number and the product of five and that number can be written algebraically as $x + 5x$.
- You may see a test question that says, "Olivia is constructing a bookcase from seven boards. Two of them are for vertical supports and five are for shelves. The height of the bookcase is twice the width of the bookcase. If the seven boards total 36 feet in length, what will be the height of Olivia's bookcase?" You would need to make a sketch and then create the equation to determine the width of the shelves. The height can be represented as double the width. (If x represents the width of the shelves in feet, then the height of the bookcase is $2x$. Since the seven boards total 36 feet, $2x + 2x + x + x + x + x + x = 36$ or $9x = 36$; $x = 4$. The height is twice the width, or 8 feet.)

Subtraction with Regrouping

A great way to make use of some of the features built into the decimal system would be regrouping when attempting longform subtraction operations. When subtracting within a place value, sometimes the minuend is smaller than the subtrahend, **regrouping** enables you to 'borrow' a unit from a place value to the left in order to get a positive difference. For example, consider subtracting 189 from 525 with regrouping.

First, set up the subtraction problem in vertical form:

$$\begin{array}{r} 525 \\ -\ 189 \\ \hline \end{array}$$

Notice that the numbers in the ones and tens columns of 525 are smaller than the numbers in the ones and tens columns of 189. This means you will need to use regrouping to perform subtraction:

$$\begin{array}{rrrr} & 5 & 2 & 5 \\ - & 1 & 8 & 9 \\ \hline \end{array}$$

To subtract 9 from 5 in the ones column you will need to borrow from the 2 in the tens columns:

$$\begin{array}{rrrr} & 5 & 1 & 15 \\ - & 1 & 8 & 9 \\ \hline & & & 6 \end{array}$$

Next, to subtract 8 from 1 in the tens column you will need to borrow from the 5 in the hundreds column:

$$\begin{array}{rrrr} & 4 & 11 & 15 \\ - & 1 & 8 & 9 \\ \hline & & 3 & 6 \end{array}$$

Mathematics

Last, subtract the 1 from the 4 in the hundreds column:

	4	11	15
-	1	8	9
	3	3	6

Review Video: Subtracting Large Numbers
Visit mometrix.com/academy and enter code: 603350

ORDER OF OPERATIONS

The **order of operations** is a set of rules that dictates the order in which we must perform each operation in an expression so that we will evaluate it accurately. If we have an expression that includes multiple different operations, the order of operations tells us which operations to do first. The most common mnemonic for the order of operations is **PEMDAS**, or "Please Excuse My Dear Aunt Sally." PEMDAS stands for parentheses, exponents, multiplication, division, addition, and subtraction. It is important to understand that multiplication and division have equal precedence, as do addition and subtraction, so those pairs of operations are simply worked from left to right in order.

For example, evaluating the expression $5 + 20 \div 4 \times (2 + 3)^2 - 6$ using the correct order of operations would be done like this:

- **P:** Perform the operations inside the parentheses: $(2 + 3) = 5$
- **E:** Simplify the exponents: $(5)^2 = 5 \times 5 = 25$
  - The expression now looks like this: $5 + 20 \div 4 \times 25 - 6$
- **MD:** Perform multiplication and division from left to right: $20 \div 4 = 5$; then $5 \times 25 = 125$
  - The expression now looks like this: $5 + 125 - 6$
- **AS:** Perform addition and subtraction from left to right: $5 + 125 = 130$; then $130 - 6 = 124$

Review Video: Order of Operations
Visit mometrix.com/academy and enter code: 259675

PROPERTIES OF OPERATIONS

THE COMMUTATIVE PROPERTY

The commutative property applies to addition and multiplication and states that these operations can be completed in any order. The **commutative property of addition** states that numbers and terms can be added together in any order to still get the same value. For example, $3 + 4 = 7$ and $4 + 3 = 7$. Also, we can use the commutative property of addition to show that $3x + 4 + 2^2$ is equivalent to $4 + 3x + 2^2$ and $2^2 + 4 + 3x$. When adding terms, you can add in any order and get the same value.

The **commutative property of multiplication** states that numbers and terms can be multiplied in any order to get the same value. For example, 12×3 is equivalent to 3×12. Additionally, we can use the commutative property of multiplication to assume that $(5 + 3) \times (36 - 6)$ is equivalent to $(36 - 6) \times (5 + 3)$. You can multiply terms in any order and still get the same value.

THE ASSOCIATIVE PROPERTY

The **associative property of addition** states that if three or more terms are being added together, the value is the same regardless of the groupings.

For example, given the expression $3 + 4 + 6$, these terms can be grouped and added in any form. $3 + 4 + 6$ is equivalent to $(3 + 4) + 6$ and is also equivalent to $3 + (4 + 6)$. This can be applied to write equivalent expressions in a variety of ways.

For example, suppose we are given the expression $5 + (y + 2) + 4$. We can generate equivalent expressions knowing the associative property. Knowing that when three or more terms are added, the grouping is irrelevant, we can say that this expression is equivalent to $5 + y + (2 + 4)$, and it is equivalent to $(5 + y) + (2 + 4)$. It is even equivalent to $5 + y + 2 + 4$.

The **associative property of multiplication** states that if three or more terms are being multiplied together, the value is the same regardless of the grouping. We can use this property to identify and generate equivalent expressions.

For example, given the expression $2 \times 7 \times 3$, these terms can be grouped in any way and still get the same value. $2 \times 7 \times 3$ is equivalent to $(2 \times 7) \times 3$ or $2 \times (7 \times 3)$.

The Identity Property

The **identity property of multiplication** states that when a number is multiplied by 1, you get the same number. That is, anything multiplied by 1 is itself. For example, $2 \times 1 = 2$, or $1 \times -36 = -36$. Using the identity property of multiplication, we can identify and generate equivalent expressions. Let's say that we are given the expression $15 - (3 \times 4)$. We can generate equivalent expressions using the identity property. One equivalent expression example would be $(15 \times 1) - (3 \times 4)$. Another example would be $15 - (1 \times 3 \times 4)$. We can say these expressions are equivalent because the identity property of multiplication states that we can multiply any portion of an expression by 1 to get the same value.

The **identity property of addition** states that when 0 is added to a number, you get the same number. For example, $2 + 0 = 2$, or $0 + -3 = -3$. We can also use this property to identify and generate equivalent expressions. For example, if we are given the expression $2 \times (1 + 2)$, we could write the equivalent expressions $2 \times (0 + 1 + 2)$ or $(2 + 0) \times (1 + 2)$.

The Inverse Property

The **inverse property of addition** states that the sum of a number and its opposite is always equal to 0. Remember, the opposite of a number is a number that is opposite on the number line from zero, or the same number with the opposite sign. For example, −4 is opposite to 4, and 1,726.9 is opposite to −1,726.9. So, the inverse property of addition states that if you add opposite numbers, their sum is zero. For example, $5 + (-5) = 0$ and $-5 + 5 = 0$.

The **inverse property of multiplication** states that a number multiplied by its reciprocal is always equal to 1. The **reciprocal** of a number is its "flipped" fraction. For example, the reciprocal of 5 is $\frac{1}{5}$, or the reciprocal of $\frac{2}{3}$ is $\frac{3}{2}$. The inverse property of multiplication can be applied for these values, $5 \times \frac{1}{5} = 1$ and $\frac{2}{3} \times \frac{3}{2} = 1$. This is because when you multiply across, you get a fraction that is equal to 1.

$$\frac{2}{3} \times \frac{3}{2} = \frac{6}{6} = 1$$

The Distributive Property

The **distributive property** explains how multiplication and addition interact. It says that when multiplying one number by the sum of two other numbers, the same result can also be obtained by

Mathematics

multiplying the one number by each of the numbers individually and then adding the products. For example, to multiply 2 by the sum of 7 and 3, the direct approach says, "the sum of 7 and 3 is 10, and 2 times 10 is 20." This would be expressed as $2 \times (7 + 3) = 2 \times 10 = 20$. On the other hand, the distributive property states that the same answer can be achieved by multiplying each number inside the parentheses and adding the products. That is, "the product of 2 and 7 is 14, the product of 2 and 3 is 6, and the sum of 14 and 6 is 20." This would be expressed as $2 \times (7 + 3) = 2 \times 7 + 2 \times 3 = 14 + 6 = 20$, and it is demonstrated below.

$$2 \times (7 + 3) = 2 \times 7 + 2 \times 3$$

This same concept can be used when multiplying a number by the difference of two numbers. For example, $5 \times (10 - 4) = 5 \times 10 - 5 \times 4$. Since $5 \times 10 = 50$ and $5 \times 4 = 20$, the result is $50 - 20 = 30$. This answer can be checked by subtracting inside the parentheses first and then multiplying: $5 \times (10 - 4) = 5 \times 6 = 30$.

> **Review Video: Commutative, Associative, and Distributive Properties**
> Visit mometrix.com/academy and enter code: 483176

PROPERTIES OF EXPONENTS

The properties of exponents are as follows:

Property	Description
$a^1 = a$	Any number to the power of 1 is equal to itself
$1^n = 1$	The number 1 raised to any power is equal to 1
$a^0 = 1$	Any number raised to the power of 0 is equal to 1
$a^n \times a^m = a^{n+m}$	Add exponents to multiply powers of the same base number
$a^n \div a^m = a^{n-m}$	Subtract exponents to divide powers of the same base number
$(a^n)^m = a^{n \times m}$	When a power is raised to a power, the exponents are multiplied
$(a \times b)^n = a^n \times b^n$ $(a \div b)^n = a^n \div b^n$	Multiplication and division operations inside parentheses can be raised to a power. This is the same as each term being raised to that power.
$a^{-n} = \frac{1}{a^n}$	A negative exponent is the same as the reciprocal of a positive exponent

Note that exponents do not have to be integers. Fractional or decimal exponents follow all the rules above as well. Example: $5^{\frac{1}{4}} \times 5^{\frac{3}{4}} = 5^{\frac{1}{4}+\frac{3}{4}} = 5^1 = 5$.

> **Review Video: Properties of Exponents**
> Visit mometrix.com/academy and enter code: 532558

SCIENTIFIC NOTATION

Scientific notation is a way of writing large numbers in a shorter form. The form $a \times 10^n$ is used in scientific notation, where a is greater than or equal to 1 but less than 10, and n is the number of places the decimal must move to get from the original number to a. Example: The number 230,400,000 is cumbersome to write. To write the value in scientific notation, place a decimal point between the first and second numbers, and include all digits through the last non-zero digit ($a = 2.304$). To find the appropriate power of 10, count the number of places the decimal point had to move ($n = 8$). The number is positive if the decimal moved to the left, and negative if it moved to the right. We can then write 230,400,000 as 2.304×10^8. If we look instead at the number 0.00002304, we have the same value for a, but this time the decimal moved 5 places to the right ($n = -5$). Thus, 0.00002304 can be written as 2.304×10^{-5}. Using this notation makes it simple to compare very large or very small numbers. By comparing exponents, it is easy to see that 3.28×10^4 is smaller than 1.51×10^5, because 4 is less than 5.

> **Review Video: Scientific Notation**
> Visit mometrix.com/academy and enter code: 976454

Factors and Multiples

Factors and Greatest Common Factor

A whole number a is a **factor** (or **divisor**) of a whole number b if a divides b evenly. In other words, a is a factor of b if the quotient $b \div a$ is a whole number with a remainder of 0. For instance, 3 is a factor of 12 because $12 \div 3 = 4$ with no remainder. Another way to say this is that a is a factor of b if we can multiply a by another whole number to get b. So, we can also show that 3 is a factor of 12 by noting that $3 \times 4 = 12$.

Every positive whole number has 1 and itself as factors. If a whole number greater than one has *only* 1 and itself as factors, we call it a **prime number**. For instance, 5 is a prime number because its only factors are 1 and 5. The first several prime numbers are 2, 3, 5, 7, 11, and 13.

If a whole number greater than 1 is not prime—that is, if it has factors besides 1 and itself—then it is a **composite number.** For instance, 10 is a composite number because it has factors 2 and 5 in addition to 1 and 10. The first several composite numbers are 4, 6, 8, 9, 10, 12, 14, and 15.

A **prime factor** of a whole number is a factor that is also a prime number. For example, the prime factors of 12 are 2 and 3. The prime factors of 15 are 3 and 5.

A **common factor** of two (or more) whole numbers is a number that is a factor of both (or all) of them. For example, the factors of 12 are $\underline{1}$, 2, $\underline{3}$, 4, 6, and 12, while the factors of 15 are $\underline{1}$, $\underline{3}$, 5, and 15. The common factors (underlined) of 12 and 15 are 1 and 3.

The **greatest common factor** (**GCF**) of two (or more) whole numbers is the largest number that is a factor of both (or all) of them. For example, the factors of 15 are $\underline{1}$, 3, $\underline{5}$, and 15; the factors of 35 are $\underline{1}$, $\underline{5}$, 7, and 35. Therefore, the greatest common factor of 15 and 35 is 5.

> **Review Video: Factors**
> Visit mometrix.com/academy and enter code: 920086
>
> **Review Video: Prime Numbers and Factorization**
> Visit mometrix.com/academy and enter code: 760669

Multiples and Least Common Multiple

A whole number b is a **multiple** of a whole number a when a is a factor of b. This means that b is the product of a and another whole number. For example, the multiples of 7 are $0 \times 7 = 0, 1 \times 7 = 7, 2 \times 7 = 14, 3 \times 7 = 21, 4 \times 7 = 28, 5 \times 7 = 35, \ldots$. Dividing 0, 7, 14, 21, 28, and 35 by 7 results in the whole numbers 0, 1, 2, 3, 4, and 5, respectively, showing that 7 is a factor of these numbers.

The least common multiple (**LCM**) of two (or more) whole numbers is the smallest number that is a multiple of both (or all) of them. For example, the multiples of 3 are 3, 6, 9, 12, 15, ...; the multiples of 5 are 5, 10, 15, 20, ... The smallest number that appears in both lists is 15, so the least common multiple of 3 and 5 is 15.

Review Video: Multiples
Visit mometrix.com/academy and enter code: 626738

Review Video: Greatest Common Factor and Least Common Multiple
Visit mometrix.com/academy and enter code: 838699

Fractions

A **fraction** is a number that is expressed as one integer written above another integer, with a dividing line between them $\left(\frac{x}{y}\right)$. It represents the **quotient** of the two numbers "x divided by y." It can also be thought of as x out of y equal parts.

The top number of a fraction is called the **numerator**, and it represents the number of parts under consideration. The 1 in $\frac{1}{4}$ means that 1 part out of the whole is being considered in the calculation. The bottom number of a fraction is called the **denominator**, and it represents the total number of equal parts. The 4 in $\frac{1}{4}$ means that the whole consists of 4 equal parts. A fraction cannot have a denominator of zero; this is referred to as "*undefined.*"

Fractions can be manipulated, without changing the value of the fraction, by multiplying or dividing (but not adding or subtracting) both the numerator and denominator by the same number. If you divide both numbers by a common factor, you are **reducing** or simplifying the fraction. Two fractions that have the same value but are expressed differently are known as **equivalent fractions**. For example, $\frac{2}{10}, \frac{3}{15}, \frac{4}{20}$, and $\frac{5}{25}$ are all equivalent fractions. They can also all be reduced or simplified to $\frac{1}{5}$.

When two fractions are manipulated so that they have the same denominator, this is known as finding a **common denominator**. The number chosen to be that common denominator should be the least common multiple of the two original denominators. Example: $\frac{3}{4}$ and $\frac{5}{6}$; the least common multiple of 4 and 6 is 12. Manipulating to achieve the common denominator: $\frac{3}{4} = \frac{9}{12}; \frac{5}{6} = \frac{10}{12}$.

Review Video: Overview of Fractions
Visit mometrix.com/academy and enter code: 262335

Proper Fractions and Mixed Numbers

A fraction whose denominator is greater than its numerator is known as a **proper fraction**, while a fraction whose numerator is greater than its denominator is known as an **improper fraction**. Proper fractions have values *less than one* and improper fractions have values *greater than one.*

A **mixed number** is a number that contains both an integer and a fraction. Any improper fraction can be rewritten as a mixed number. Example: $\frac{8}{3} = \frac{6}{3} + \frac{2}{3} = 2 + \frac{2}{3} = 2\frac{2}{3}$. Similarly, any mixed number can be rewritten as an improper fraction. Example: $1\frac{3}{5} = 1 + \frac{3}{5} = \frac{5}{5} + \frac{3}{5} = \frac{8}{5}$.

Review Video: Proper and Improper Fractions and Mixed Numbers
Visit mometrix.com/academy and enter code: 211077

Adding and Subtracting Fractions

If two fractions have a common denominator, they can be added or subtracted simply by adding or subtracting the two numerators and retaining the same denominator. If the two fractions do not already have the same denominator, one or both of them must be manipulated to achieve a common denominator before they can be added or subtracted. Example: $\frac{1}{2} + \frac{1}{4} = \frac{2}{4} + \frac{1}{4} = \frac{3}{4}$.

Review Video: Adding and Subtracting Fractions
Visit mometrix.com/academy and enter code: 378080

Multiplying Fractions

Two fractions can be multiplied by multiplying the two numerators to find the new numerator and the two denominators to find the new denominator. Example: $\frac{1}{3} \times \frac{2}{3} = \frac{1\times 2}{3\times 3} = \frac{2}{9}$.

Dividing Fractions

Two fractions can be divided by flipping the numerator and denominator of the second fraction and then proceeding as though it were a multiplication problem. Example: $\frac{2}{3} \div \frac{3}{4} = \frac{2}{3} \times \frac{4}{3} = \frac{8}{9}$.

Review Video: Multiplying and Dividing Fractions
Visit mometrix.com/academy and enter code: 473632

Multiplying a Mixed Number by a Whole Number or a Decimal

When multiplying a mixed number by something, it is usually best to convert it to an improper fraction first. Additionally, if the multiplicand is a decimal, it is most often simplest to convert it to a fraction. For instance, to multiply $4\frac{3}{8}$ by 3.5, begin by rewriting each quantity as a whole number plus a proper fraction. Remember, a mixed number is a fraction added to a whole number and a decimal is a representation of the sum of fractions, specifically tenths, hundredths, thousandths, and so on:

$$4\frac{3}{8} \times 3.5 = \left(4 + \frac{3}{8}\right) \times \left(3 + \frac{1}{2}\right)$$

Next, the quantities being added need to be expressed with the same denominator. This is achieved by multiplying and dividing the whole number by the denominator of the fraction. Recall that a whole number is equivalent to that number divided by 1:

$$= \left(\frac{4}{1} \times \frac{8}{8} + \frac{3}{8}\right) \times \left(\frac{3}{1} \times \frac{2}{2} + \frac{1}{2}\right)$$

Mathematics

When multiplying fractions, remember to multiply the numerators and denominators separately:

$$= \left(\frac{4 \times 8}{1 \times 8} + \frac{3}{8}\right) \times \left(\frac{3 \times 2}{1 \times 2} + \frac{1}{2}\right)$$
$$= \left(\frac{32}{8} + \frac{3}{8}\right) \times \left(\frac{6}{2} + \frac{1}{2}\right)$$

Now that the fractions have the same denominators, they can be added:

$$= \frac{35}{8} \times \frac{7}{2}$$

Finally, perform the last multiplication and then simplify:

$$= \frac{35 \times 7}{8 \times 2} = \frac{245}{16} = \frac{240}{16} + \frac{5}{16} = 15\frac{5}{16}$$

Comparing Fractions

It is important to master the ability to compare and order fractions. This skill is relevant to many real-world scenarios. For example, carpenters often compare fractional construction nail lengths when preparing for a project, and bakers often compare fractional measurements to have the correct ratio of ingredients. There are three commonly used strategies when comparing fractions. These strategies are referred to as the common denominator approach, the decimal approach, and the cross-multiplication approach.

Using a Common Denominator to Compare Fractions

The fractions $\frac{2}{3}$ and $\frac{4}{7}$ have different denominators. $\frac{2}{3}$ has a denominator of 3, and $\frac{4}{7}$ has a denominator of 7. In order to precisely compare these two fractions, it is necessary to use a common denominator. A common denominator is a common multiple that is shared by both denominators. In this case, the denominators 3 and 7 share a multiple of 21. In general, it is most efficient to select the least common multiple for the two denominators.

Rewrite each fraction with the common denominator of 21. Then, calculate the new numerators as illustrated below.

$$\frac{2}{3} \xrightarrow{\times 7} \frac{\mathbf{14}}{21} \qquad \frac{4}{7} \xrightarrow{\times 3} \frac{\mathbf{12}}{21}$$

For $\frac{2}{3}$, multiply the numerator and denominator by 7. The result is $\frac{14}{21}$.

For $\frac{4}{7}$, multiply the numerator and denominator by 3. The result is $\frac{12}{21}$.

Now that both fractions have a denominator of 21, the fractions can accurately be compared by comparing the numerators. Since 14 is greater than 12, the fraction $\frac{14}{21}$ is greater than $\frac{12}{21}$. This means that $\frac{2}{3}$ is greater than $\frac{4}{7}$.

Using Decimals to Compare Fractions

Sometimes decimal values are easier to compare than fraction values. For example, $\frac{5}{8}$ is equivalent to 0.625 and $\frac{3}{5}$ is equivalent to 0.6. This means that the comparison of $\frac{5}{8}$ and $\frac{3}{5}$ can be determined by comparing the decimals 0.625 and 0.6. When both decimal values are extended to the thousandths place, they become 0.625 and 0.600, respectively. It becomes clear that 0.625 is greater than 0.600 because 625 thousandths is greater than 600 thousandths. In other words, $\frac{5}{8}$ is greater than $\frac{3}{5}$ because 0.625 is greater than 0.6.

Using Cross-Multiplication to Compare Fractions

Cross-multiplication is an efficient strategy for comparing fractions. This is a shortcut for the common denominator strategy. Start by writing each fraction next to one another. Multiply the numerator of the fraction on the left by the denominator of the fraction on the right. Write down the result next to the fraction on the left. Now multiply the numerator of the fraction on the right by the denominator of the fraction on the left. Write down the result next to the fraction on the right. Compare both products. The fraction with the larger result is the larger fraction.

Consider the fractions $\frac{4}{7}$ and $\frac{5}{9}$.

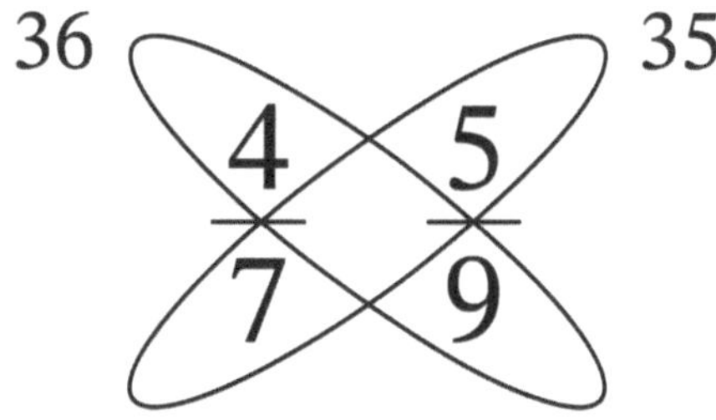

36 is greater than 35. Therefore, $\frac{4}{7}$ is greater than $\frac{5}{9}$.

Decimals

Decimals are one way to represent parts of a whole. Using the place value system, each digit to the right of a decimal point denotes the number of units of a corresponding *negative* power of ten. For example, consider the decimal 0.24. We can use a model to represent the decimal. Since a dime is worth one-tenth of a dollar and a penny is worth one-hundredth of a dollar, one possible model to represent this fraction is to have 2 dimes representing the 2 in the tenths place and 4 pennies representing the 4 in the hundredths place:

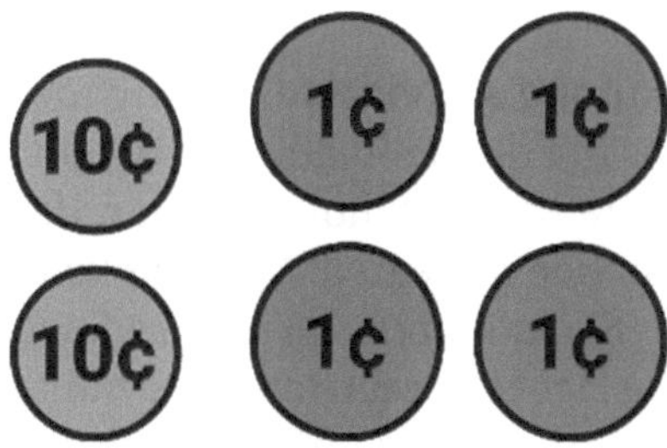

To write the decimal as a fraction, put the decimal in the numerator with 1 in the denominator. Multiply the numerator and denominator by tens until there are no more decimal places. Then simplify the fraction to lowest terms. For example, converting 0.24 to a fraction:

$$0.24 = \frac{0.24}{1} = \frac{0.24 \times 100}{1 \times 100} = \frac{24}{100} = \frac{6}{25}$$

Review Video: Decimals
Visit mometrix.com/academy and enter code: 837268

Operations with Decimals

Adding and Subtracting Decimals

When adding and subtracting decimals, the decimal points must always be aligned. Adding decimals is just like adding regular whole numbers. Example: $4.5 + 2.0 = 6.5$.

If the problem-solver does not properly align the decimal points, an incorrect answer of 4.7 may result. An easy way to add decimals is to align all of the decimal points in a vertical column visually. This will allow you to see exactly where the decimal should be placed in the final answer. Begin adding from right to left. Add each column in turn, making sure to carry the number to the left if a column adds up to more than 9. The same rules apply to the subtraction of decimals.

Review Video: Adding and Subtracting Decimals
Visit mometrix.com/academy and enter code: 381101

Multiplying Decimals

A simple multiplication problem has two components: a **multiplicand** and a **multiplier**. When multiplying decimals, work as though the numbers were whole rather than decimals. Once the final product is calculated, count the number of places to the right of the decimal in both the multiplicand and the multiplier. Then, count that number of places from the right of the product and place the decimal in that position.

For example, 12.3×2.56 has a total of three places to the right of the respective decimals. Multiply 123×256 to get 31,488. Now, beginning on the right, count three places to the left and insert the decimal. The final product will be 31.488.

Review Video: How to Multiply Decimals
Visit mometrix.com/academy and enter code: 731574

Dividing Decimals

Every division problem has a **divisor** and a **dividend**. The dividend is the number that is being divided. In the problem $14 \div 7$, 14 is the dividend and 7 is the divisor. In a division problem with decimals, the divisor must be converted into a whole number. Begin by moving the decimal in the divisor to the right until a whole number is created. Next, move the decimal in the dividend the same number of spaces to the right. For example, 4.9 into 24.5 would become 49 into 245. The decimal was moved one space to the right to create a whole number in the divisor, and then the same was done for the dividend. Once the whole numbers are created, the problem is carried out normally: $245 \div 49 = 5$.

Review Video: Dividing Decimals
Visit mometrix.com/academy and enter code: 560690

Review Video: Dividing Decimals by Whole Numbers
Visit mometrix.com/academy and enter code: 535669

PERCENTAGES

Percentages can be thought of as fractions that are based on a whole of 100; that is, one whole is equal to 100%. The word **percent** means "per hundred." Percentage problems are often presented in three main ways:

- Find what percentage of some number another number is.
  - Example: What percentage of 40 is 8?
- Find what number is some percentage of a given number.
  - Example: What number is 20% of 40?
- Find what number another number is a given percentage of.
  - Example: What number is 8 20% of?

There are three components in each of these cases: a **whole** (W), a **part** (P), and a **percentage** (%). These are related by the equation: $P = W \times \%$. This can easily be rearranged into other forms that may suit different questions better: $\% = \frac{P}{W}$ and $W = \frac{P}{\%}$. Percentage problems are often also word problems. As such, a large part of solving them is figuring out which quantities are what. For example, consider the following word problem:

In a school cafeteria, 7 students choose pizza, 9 choose hamburgers, and 4 choose tacos. What percentage of student choose tacos?

To find the whole, you must first add all of the parts: $7 + 9 + 4 = 20$. The percentage can then be found by dividing the part by the whole $\left(\% = \frac{P}{W}\right)$: $\frac{4}{20} = \frac{20}{100} = 20\%$.

Review Video: Computation with Percentages
Visit mometrix.com/academy and enter code: 693099

CALCULATING PERCENT CHANGE

Suppose a quantity has a particular value (the *old value*) and then we add something (the *change*) to it to get another value (the *new value*). We can describe this process by the simple equation (old value) + change = (new value). If we know the old and new values, we can rearrange this equation to find the change, getting change = (new value) − (old value). For instance, if a store's price for a box of computer paper goes from \$20 last week to \$25 this week, this is a change of (new value) − (old value) = \$25 − \$20 = \$5. Or, if the size of the freshman class at a college goes from 500 students one year to 440 students the next year, this is a change of (new value) − (old value) = 440 − 500 = −60 students. So, we see that change can be positive or negative.

Instead of the word *change*, we sometimes use the words *increase* or *decrease* to specify whether the value goes up or down, respectively. In the examples above, the price of computer paper increases by \$5 and the freshman class decreases by 60 students. Note that the decrease is 60 students and not -60 because the word *decrease* already means that the value goes down. So, *increase* is the same as positive change and *decrease* is the opposite or negative change.

If the changing quantity represents an amount (how much of something there is), we can also calculate the **percent change**. This is the change expressed as a percentage of the old amount. To calculate this, we divide the change by the old amount and express the quotient as a percent. That is, we use the formula percent change $= \frac{\text{change}}{\text{old value}}$, converting the resulting decimal answer to a percent. In the examples above, the price of a box of computer paper has a percent change of $\frac{\text{change in price}}{\text{old price}} = \frac{\$5}{\$20} = 0.25 = 25\%$, and the size of the freshman class at the college has a percent change of $\frac{\text{change in enrollment}}{\text{old enrollment}} = \frac{-60}{500} = -0.12 = -12\%$. We can also use the terms *percent increase* and *percent decrease*, saying that the price of computer paper increases by 25% and the size of the freshman class decreases by 12%. Note that the denominator is always the old amount, never the new amount.

Example: Your landlord raises your rent from $1,500 to $1,700 per month. To find the percent change in your rent (rounded to the nearest tenth of a percent), you calculate as follows.

$$\begin{aligned}\text{percent change in rent} &= \frac{\text{change in rent}}{\text{old rent}} = \frac{(\text{new rent}) - (\text{old rent})}{\text{old rent}} \\ &= \frac{\$1{,}700 - \$1{,}500}{\$1{,}500} = \frac{\$200}{\$1{,}500} = 0.1333\ldots \approx 13.3\%\end{aligned}$$

Therefore, the percent change in your rent is approximately 13.3%.

Review Video: Percent Change
Visit mometrix.com/academy and enter code: 907890

Converting Between Percentages, Fractions, and Decimals

Converting decimals to percentages and percentages to decimals is as simple as moving the decimal point. To *convert from a decimal to a percentage*, move the decimal point **two places to the right**. To *convert from a percentage to a decimal*, move it **two places to the left**. It may be helpful to remember that the percentage number will always be larger than the equivalent decimal number. Example:

$$\begin{array}{lll} 0.23 = 23\% & 5.34 = 534\% & 0.007 = 0.7\% \\ 700\% = 7.00 & 86\% = 0.86 & 0.15\% = 0.0015 \end{array}$$

To convert a fraction to a decimal, simply divide the numerator by the denominator in the fraction. To convert a decimal to a fraction, put the decimal in the numerator with 1 in the denominator. Multiply the numerator and denominator by tens until there are no more decimal places. Then simplify the fraction to lowest terms. For example, converting 0.24 to a fraction:

$$0.24 = \frac{0.24}{1} = \frac{0.24 \times 100}{1 \times 100} = \frac{24}{100} = \frac{6}{25}$$

Fractions can be converted to a percentage by finding equivalent fractions with a denominator of 100. Example:

$$\frac{7}{10} = \frac{70}{100} = 70\% \quad \frac{1}{4} = \frac{25}{100} = 25\%$$

To convert a percentage to a fraction, divide the percentage number by 100 and reduce the fraction to its simplest possible terms. Example:

$$60\% = \frac{60}{100} = \frac{3}{5} \quad 96\% = \frac{96}{100} = \frac{24}{25}$$

Review Video: Converting Fractions to Percentages and Decimals
Visit mometrix.com/academy and enter code: 306233

Review Video: Converting Percentages to Decimals and Fractions
Visit mometrix.com/academy and enter code: 287297

Review Video: Converting Decimals to Fractions and Percentages
Visit mometrix.com/academy and enter code: 986765

Review Video: Converting Decimals, Improper Fractions, and Mixed Numbers
Visit mometrix.com/academy and enter code: 696924

Proportions and Ratios

Proportions

There is a **proportion** between two variable quantities if there is a constant relationship between their products or quotients, a relationship that does not change as the quantities themselves change.

Given variable quantities x and y, we say that they are **directly proportional** (or that y **varies directly with** x) if their quotient or *ratio* is constant—that is, if there is a constant k such that $\frac{y}{x} = k$ is always true. Another way of saying this is that y is a constant multiple of x, so that $y = kx$ is always true. We call the number k the **constant of proportionality**. For example, if you drive at a constant 50 miles per hour, then the distance, y, that you travel in miles is 50 times the number of hours, x, that you drive. In symbols, $y = 50x$ miles (or $\frac{y}{x} = 50$ mph). So, the distance you travel, y, is directly proportional to (or varies directly with) the time you travel, x, with constant of proportionality $k = 50$ mph.

The quantities x and y are **inversely proportional** (or y varies inversely with x) if their product is constant—that is, if there is a constant k such that $xy = k$ is always true. Another way of saying this is to say that y is a constant multiple of the reciprocal of x so that $y = \frac{k}{x}$ is always true. For instance, suppose you drive at speed (rate) y mph for x hours, going a total of 120 miles. Since rate × time = distance, we get $xy = 120$ miles (or $y = \frac{120}{x}$ miles per hour). Thus, your driving speed, y, is inversely proportional to (or varies inversely with) your drive time, x, with constant of proportionality $k = 120$ miles.

Review Video: Proportions
Visit mometrix.com/academy and enter code: 505355

RATIOS

A **ratio** expresses the sizes of two quantities relative to each other. For instance, suppose we have 3 copies of sheet music to share among 6 singers. We can divide the singers into groups of 2 and give each group 1 copy of the music. Thus, there is 1 copy of the music for every 2 singers, and we say that the **ratio** of sheet music to singers is 1 to 2, which we write either as a fraction $\frac{1}{2}$ or using a colon $1 : 2$. Of course, it is also true there are 3 copies for every 6 singers so that the ratio of sheet music to singers is also 3 to 6, which we write as $\frac{3}{6}$ or $3 : 6$. So, the ratios $\frac{1}{2}$ and $\frac{3}{6}$ express the same relative quantities of music and singers. We say that these ratios are equal or **equivalent**, and we note that ratios are equal precisely when their fractions are equal (so, in this case, $\frac{1}{2} = \frac{3}{6}$ as fractions). We can also express the quantities in the other order and say that the ratio of singers to music is $\frac{2}{1}$ or $2 : 1$ (or $\frac{6}{3}$ or $6 : 3$).

> **Review Video: Ratios**
> Visit mometrix.com/academy and enter code: 996914

CONSTANT OF PROPORTIONALITY

If variable quantities x and y are proportional and we know a pair of corresponding values for them, then we can find their constant of proportionality. If they are directly proportional, we use the formula $\frac{y}{x} = k$. If they are inversely proportional, we use the formula $xy = k$

Example: The cost in dollars, y, of buying fence posts is directly proportional to the number, x, that you buy. If it costs \$51 to buy 17 fence posts, what is the constant of proportionality? Because of direct proportionality, we know that $\frac{y}{x} = k$. Since this works for every pair of corresponding x- and y-values, it also works for $x = 17$ and $y = 51$. This gives us $\frac{51}{17} = k$, which simplifies to $k = 3$. Note also that this is the unit price, namely \$3 per fence post.

WORK/UNIT RATE

Unit rate expresses a quantity of one thing in terms of one unit of another. For example, if you travel 30 miles every two hours, a unit rate expresses this comparison in terms of one hour: in one hour you travel 15 miles, so your unit rate is 15 miles per hour. Other examples are how much one ounce of food costs (price per ounce) or figuring out how much one egg costs out of the dozen (price per 1 egg, instead of price per 12 eggs). The denominator of a unit rate is always 1. Unit rates are used to compare different situations to solve problems. For example, to make sure you get the best deal when deciding which kind of soda to buy, you can find the unit rate of each. If soda #1 costs \$1.50 for a 1-liter bottle, and soda #2 costs \$2.75 for a 2-liter bottle, it would be a better deal to buy soda #2, because its unit rate is only \$1.375 per 1-liter, which is cheaper than soda #1. Unit rates can also help determine the length of time a given event will take. For example, if you can paint 2 rooms in 4.5 hours, you can determine how long it will take you to paint 5 rooms by solving for the unit rate per room and then multiplying that by 5.

> **Review Video: Rates and Unit Rates**
> Visit mometrix.com/academy and enter code: 185363

Equations and Expressions

Cross Multiplication

Finding an Unknown in Equivalent Expressions

It is often necessary to apply information given about a rate or proportion to a new scenario. For example, if you know that Jedha can run a marathon (26.2 miles) in 3 hours, how long would it take her to run 10 miles at the same pace? Start by setting up equivalent expressions:

$$\frac{26.2 \text{ mi}}{3 \text{ hr}} = \frac{10 \text{ mi}}{x \text{ hr}}$$

Now, cross multiply and solve for x:

$$26.2x = 30$$
$$x = \frac{30}{26.2} = \frac{15}{13.1}$$
$$x \approx 1.15 \text{ hrs } or \text{ 1 hr 9 min}$$

So, at this pace, Jedha could run 10 miles in about 1.15 hours or about 1 hour and 9 minutes.

Review Video: Cross Multiplying Fractions
Visit mometrix.com/academy and enter code: 893904

Linear Expressions

Terms and Coefficients

Mathematical expressions consist of a combination of one or more values arranged in terms that are added together. As such, an expression could be just a single number, including zero. A **variable term** is the product of a real number, also called a **coefficient**, and one or more variables, each of which may be raised to an exponent. Expressions may also include numbers without a variable, called **constants** or **constant terms**. The expression $6s^2$, for example, is a single term where the coefficient is the real number 6 and the variable term is s^2. Note that if a term is written as simply a variable to some exponent, like t^2, then the coefficient is 1, because $t^2 = 1t^2$.

Linear Expressions

A **single variable linear expression** is the sum of a single variable term, where the variable has no exponent, and a constant, which may be zero. For instance, the expression $2w + 7$ has $2w$ as the variable term and 7 as the constant term. It is important to realize that terms are separated by addition or subtraction. Since an expression is a sum of terms, expressions such as $5x - 3$ can be written as $5x + (-3)$ to emphasize that the constant term is negative. A real-world example of a single variable linear expression is the perimeter of a square, four times the side length, often expressed: $4s$.

In general, a **linear expression** is the sum of any number of variable terms so long as none of the variables have an exponent and none of the terms have two variables multiplied together. For example, $3m + 8n - \frac{1}{4}p + 5.5q - 1$ is a linear expression, but $3y^3$ and $5xy$ are not. In the same way, the expression for the perimeter of a general triangle $(a + b + c)$ is linear, but the expression for the area of a square (s^2) is not.

Mathematics

SLOPE

FINDING SLOPE GIVEN GRAPH OR TABLE

On a graph with two points, (x_1, y_1) and (x_2, y_2), the **slope** is found with the formula $m = \frac{y_2 - y_1}{x_2 - x_1}$; where $x_1 \neq x_2$ and m stands for slope. If the value of the slope is **positive**, the line has an *upward direction* from left to right. If the value of the slope is **negative**, the line has a *downward direction* from left to right. Consider the following example:

A new book goes on sale in bookstores and online stores. In the first month, 5,000 copies of the book are sold. Over time, the book continues to grow in popularity. The data for the number of copies sold is in the table below.

# of Months on Sale	1	2	3	4	5
# of Copies Sold (In Thousands)	5	10	15	20	25

So, the number of copies that are sold and the time that the book is on sale is a proportional relationship. In this example, an equation can be used to show the data: $y = 5x$, where x is the number of months that the book is on sale. Also, y is the number of copies sold. So, the slope of the corresponding line is $\frac{\text{rise}}{\text{run}} = \frac{5}{1} = 5$.

FINDING SLOPE GIVEN AN EQUATION

When given an equation of a line, it is necessary to solve for y to determine the slope of the line. Given the equation $6x + 2y = 8$, find the slope. First, subtract $6x$ from both sides of the equation, resulting in $2y = -6x + 8$. Then divide both sides of the equation by 2, resulting in $y = -3x + 4$. This then allows us to conclude that the slope of the line is $m = -3$, the coefficient of x. Once an equation is in the form $y = mx + b$, the slope and y-intercept can easily be determined. For this reason, we refer to the equation $y = mx + b$ as "slope-intercept form" of the equation of a line.

Review Video: Finding the Slope of a Line
Visit mometrix.com/academy and enter code: 766664

LINEAR EQUATIONS

Equations like $5x = 100$ and $8x - 120 = 200$ and $6x + 4y = 240$ are **linear equations**. Linear equations are named based off the number of distinct variables they include. For example, the equation $3x + 30 = 8x$ is a **one-variable linear equation** because it involves only the single variable x. It does not matter that x appears more than once. Any equations that can be written as $ax + b = 0$, where $a \neq 0$, falls into this category. Furthermore, the equation $3x - 5y = 14 + 9y$ is a **two-variable linear equation** because it involves the two variables x and y. The equation $7x + 8y - 12z + 14w = 56$ is a linear equation in four variables.

SATISFYING THE EQUATION

When given a one-variable linear equation, the goal is typically to solve it. This means that we want to find the number that makes the equation true if we substitute it for the variable. That number is the **solution,** or root, of the equation. For instance, the equation $5x = 10$ has the solution $x = 2$. This is true because when 2 is substituted for x, the result is $5 \cdot 2 = 10$, which is true. On the other hand, $x = 6$ can not be a solution because $5 \cdot 6 \neq 10$, so it is false. Two equations with the same solution are **equivalent equations.** For example, the equations $5x = 10$ and $5x + 3 = 13$ are equivalent because both have the same solution of $x = 2$.

Determining a Solution Set

The **solution set** is the set of all solutions of an equation. In the previous example, the solution set would be 2. Solutions to a linear equation in two variables consist of pairs of numbers. For instance, the equation $6x + 4y = 240$ has the solution $x = 20$ and $y = 30$ since $6 \cdot 20 + 4 \cdot 30 = 240$ is true. We can write this solution as the ordered pair (20,30) and plot it as a point on the coordinate plane. Such equations usually have infinitely many solutions; and if we plot the points for all these solutions we get a line, which is a picture of all the solutions. We call this **graphing the equation**. When an equation has no true solutions, it is referred to as an **empty set**.

Linear Equation Forms

Linear equations can be written many ways. Below is a list of some forms linear equations can take:

- **Standard Form**: $Ax + By = C$; the slope is $\frac{-A}{B}$ and the y-intercept is $\frac{C}{B}$
- **Slope Intercept Form**: $y = mx + b$, where m is the slope and b is the y-intercept
- **Point-Slope Form**: $y - y_1 = m(x - x_1)$, where m is the slope and (x_1, y_1) is a point on the line
- **Two-Point Form**: $\frac{y-y_1}{x-x_1} = \frac{y_2-y_1}{x_2-x_1}$, where (x_1, y_1) and (x_2, y_2) are two points on the given line
- **Intercept Form**: $\frac{x}{x_1} + \frac{y}{y_1} = 1$, where $(x_1, 0)$ is the point at which a line intersects the x-axis, and $(0, y_1)$ is the point at which the same line intersects the y-axis

Review Video: Slope-Intercept and Point-Slope Forms
Visit mometrix.com/academy and enter code: 113216

Review Video: Converting Between Standard and Slope-Intercept Forms
Visit mometrix.com/academy and enter code: 982828

Review Video: Linear Equations Basics
Visit mometrix.com/academy and enter code: 793005

Solving Equations

Manipulating Equations

Like Terms

Like terms are terms in an equation that have the same variable, regardless of whether they also have the same coefficient. This includes terms that *lack* a variable; all constants (i.e., numbers without variables) are considered like terms. If the equation involves terms with a variable raised to different powers, the like terms are those that have the variable raised to the same power.

For example, consider the equation $x^2 + 3x + 2 = 2x^2 + x - 7 + 2x$. In this equation, 2 and –7 are like terms; they are both constants. The terms $3x$, x, and $2x$ are like terms, they all include the variable x raised to the first power. The terms x^2 and $2x^2$ are like terms, they both include the variable x, raised to the second power. The terms $2x$ and $2x^2$ are not like terms; although they both involve the variable x, the variable is not raised to the same power in both terms. The fact that they have the same coefficient, 2, is not relevant.

Review Video: Rules for Manipulating Equations
Visit mometrix.com/academy and enter code: 838871

Carrying Out the Same Operation on Both Sides of an Equation

When solving an equation, the general procedure is to carry out a series of operations on both sides of an equation, choosing operations that simplify the equation when doing so. The reason why the same operation must be carried out on both sides of the equation is because that leaves the meaning of the equation unchanged, and yields a result that is equivalent to the original equation. This would not be the case if we carried out an operation on one side of an equation and not the other. Consider what an equation means: it is a statement that two values or expressions are equal. If we carry out the same operation on both sides of the equation—add 3 to both sides, for example—then the two sides of the equation are changed in the same way, and so remain equal. If we do that to only one side of the equation—add 3 to one side but not the other—then that wouldn't be true; if we change one side of the equation but not the other then the two sides are no longer equal.

Combining Like Terms

Combining like terms refers to adding or subtracting like terms—terms with the same variable—and therefore reducing sets of like terms to a single term. The main advantage of doing this is that it simplifies the equation. Often, combining like terms can be done as the first step in solving an equation, though it can also be done later, such as after distributing terms in a product.

For example, consider the equation $2(x + 3) + 3(2 + x + 3) = -4$. The 2 and the 3 in the second set of parentheses are like terms, and we can combine them, yielding $2(x + 3) + 3(x + 5) = -4$. Now we can carry out the multiplications implied by the parentheses, distributing the outer 2 and 3 accordingly: $2x + 6 + 3x + 15 = -4$. The $2x$ and the $3x$ are like terms, and we can add them together: $5x + 6 + 15 = -4$. Now, the constants 6, 15, and -4 are also like terms, and we can combine them as well: subtracting 6 and 15 from both sides of the equation, we get $5x = -4 - 6 - 15$, or $5x = -25$, which simplifies further to $x = -5$.

Review Video: Solving Equations by Combining Like Terms
Visit mometrix.com/academy and enter code: 668506

Canceling Terms on Opposite Sides of an Equation

Two terms on opposite sides of an equation can be canceled if and only if they *exactly* match each other. They must have the same variable raised to the same power and the same coefficient. For example, in the equation $3x + 2x^2 + 6 = 2x^2 - 6$, $2x^2$ appears on both sides of the equation and can be canceled, leaving $3x + 6 = -6$. The 6 on each side of the equation *cannot* be canceled, because it is added on one side of the equation and subtracted on the other. While they cannot be canceled, however, the 6 and -6 are like terms and can be combined, yielding $3x = -12$, which simplifies further to $x = -4$.

It's also important to note that the terms to be canceled must be independent terms and cannot be part of a larger term. For example, consider the equation $2(x + 6) = 3(x + 4) + 1$. We cannot cancel the x's, because even though they match each other they are part of the larger terms $2(x + 6)$ and $3(x + 4)$. We must first distribute the 2 and 3, yielding $2x + 12 = 3x + 12 + 1$. Now we see that the terms with the x's do not match, but the 12s do, and can be canceled, leaving $2x = 3x + 1$, which simplifies to $x = -1$.

Isolating Variables

To isolate a variable means to manipulate the equation so that the variable appears by itself on one side of the equation, and does not appear at all on the other side. Generally, an equation or inequality is considered to be solved once the variable is isolated and the other side of the equation or inequality is simplified as much as possible. In the case of a two-variable equation or inequality, only one variable needs to be isolated; it will not usually be possible to simultaneously isolate both variables.

For a linear equation—an equation in which the variable only appears raised to the first power—isolating a variable can be done by first moving all the terms with the variable to one side of the equation and all other terms to the other side. (*Moving* a term really means adding the inverse of the term to both sides; when a term is *moved* to the other side of the equation its sign is flipped.) Then combine like terms on each side. Finally, divide both sides by the coefficient of the variable, if applicable. The steps need not necessarily be done in this order, but this order will always work.

Review Video: Solving Equations for Specific Variables
Visit mometrix.com/academy and enter code: 130695

Review Video: Solving Equations Involving Algebraic Fractions
Visit mometrix.com/academy and enter code: 237770

Review Video: Solving One-Step Equations
Visit mometrix.com/academy and enter code: 777004

SOLVING ONE-VARIABLE LINEAR EQUATIONS

EQUATIONS WITH ONE SOLUTION (THE USUAL CASE)

To solve a one-variable linear equation, we use the techniques above to isolate the variable.

1. If any coefficients or constants are fractions, it is often helpful first to multiply both sides of the equation by the least common denominator (of all fractions) to clear the fractions.
2. Simplify both sides of the equation by combining any like terms.
3. Put all terms with the variable on one side of the equation and all constant terms on the other side, by adding or subtracting the same terms on both sides of the equation.
4. Divide both sides by the coefficient of the variable (or multiply both sides by its reciprocal).
5. When we have a value for the variable, we can check it by substituting the value into the original equation to make sure it produces a true result.

Consider the following example for solving the equation $\frac{2}{3}x + 8 = 14$:

$3 \cdot \left(\frac{2}{3}x + 8\right) = 3 \cdot 14$	Clear fractions by multiplying both sides by 3.
$2x + 24 = 42$	Simplify, remembering to apply the distributive property.
$2x + 24 - 24 = 42 - 24$	Subtract 24 from both sides to isolate $2x$.
$2x = 18$	Simplify by combining like terms.
$\frac{2x}{2} = \frac{18}{2}$	Divide both sides by 2 to isolate x.
$x = 9$	Simplify

Mathematics

Finally, we check this answer by substituting $x = 9$ into the original equation to make sure we get a true result.

$$\frac{2}{3}x + 8 = \frac{2}{3}(9) + 8 = 6 + 8 = 14$$

This is correct, so the value of x is 9.

Review Video: Solving Equations Using the Distributive Property
Visit mometrix.com/academy and enter code: 765499

Equations with More Than One Solution

Some types of non-linear equations, such as equations involving squares of variables, may have more than one solution. For example, the equation $x^2 = 4$ has two solutions: 2 and –2. Equations with absolute values can also have multiple solutions: $|x| = 1$ has the solutions $x = 1$ and $x = -1$.

It is possible for a linear equation to have more than one solution but only if the equation is true regardless of the value of the variable. We call such an equation an **identity**. In this case, the equation has infinitely many solutions, because every possible value of the variable is a solution. We discover that a linear equation is an identity when our attempts to isolate the variable cause the variable to disappear, leaving a *true* equation involving only constants. For example, consider the equation $2(3x + 5) = x + 5(x + 2)$. Distributing, we get $6x + 10 = x + 5x + 10$; combining like terms gives $6x + 10 = 6x + 10$, and the $6x$-terms cancel to leave $10 = 10$. This is clearly true, so the original equation is an identity. We could also cancel the 10's leaving $0 = 0$, which is also is clearly true—in general if both sides of the equation can be reduced to match one another exactly, the original equation is an identity.

Equations with No Solution

Some types of non-linear equations, such as equations involving squares of variables, may have no solution. For example, the equation $x^2 = -2$ has no solutions in the real numbers because the square of a real number must be positive. Similarly, $|x| = -1$ has no solution because the absolute value of a number is always positive.

It is also possible for a linear equation to have no solution. We call such an equation a **contradiction**. We discover that a linear equation is a contradiction when our attempts to isolate the variable cause the variable to disappear, leaving a *false* equation involving only constants. For example, the equation $2(x + 3) + x = 3x$ has no solution. We can see this by trying to solve it: first we distribute, leaving $2x + 6 + x = 3x$. Combining like terms gives us $3x + 6 = 3x$, and cancelling the term $3x$ on both sides leaves us with $6 = 0$. This is clearly false, so the original equation is a contradiction, having no solutions.

Features of Equations That Require Special Treatment

A linear equation is an equation in which variables only appear by themselves: not multiplied together, not with exponents other than one, and not inside absolute value signs or any other functions. For example, the equation $x + 1 - 3x = 5 - x$ is a linear equation; while x appears multiple times, it never appears with an exponent other than one, or inside any function. The two-variable equation $2x - 3y = 5 + 2x$ is also a linear equation. In contrast, the equation $x^2 - 5 = 3x$ is *not* a linear equation, because it involves the term x^2. The equation $\sqrt{x} = 5$ is not linear, because it involves a square root. The equation $(x - 1)^2 = 4$ is not linear because even though there's no exponent on the x directly, it appears as part of an expression that is squared. The two-variable equation $x + xy - y = 5$ is not linear because it includes the term xy, where two variables are multiplied together.

As we see above, linear equations can always be solved (or shown to have no solution) by combining like terms and performing simple operations on both sides of the equation. Some non-linear equations can be solved by similar methods, but others may require more advanced methods of solution, if they can be solved analytically at all.

Solving Equations Involving Roots

In an equation involving roots, the first step is to isolate the term with the root, if possible, and then raise both sides of the equation to the appropriate power to eliminate it. Consider an example equation, $2\sqrt{x+1} - 1 = 3$. In this case, begin by adding 1 to both sides, yielding $2\sqrt{x+1} = 4$, and then dividing both sides by 2, yielding $\sqrt{x+1} = 2$. Now square both sides, yielding $x + 1 = 4$. Finally, subtracting 1 from both sides yields $x = 3$.

Squaring both sides of an equation (or raising both sides to any *even* power) may, however, yield a spurious solution—a solution to the squared equation that is *not* a solution of the original equation. It's therefore necessary to plug the solution back into the original equation to make sure it works. In this case, it does: $2\sqrt{3+1} - 1 = 2\sqrt{4} - 1 = 2(2) - 1 = 4 - 1 = 3$.

The same procedure applies for other roots as well. For example, given the equation $3 + \sqrt[3]{2x} = 5$, we can first subtract 3 from both sides, yielding $\sqrt[3]{2x} = 2$ and isolating the root. Raising both sides to the third power yields $2x = 2^3$; i.e., $2x = 8$. We can now divide both sides by 2 to get $x = 4$.

> **Review Video: Solving Equations Involving Roots**
> Visit mometrix.com/academy and enter code: 297670

Solving Equations with Exponents

In solving an equation with powers of a variable, sometimes it is possible to eliminate all but one term involving the variable. In that case, we can isolate the power of the variable and then take the appropriate root of both sides to eliminate the exponent. For instance, for the equation $2x^3 + 17 = 5x^3 - 7$, we can subtract $5x^3$ from both sides to get $-3x^3 + 17 = -7$, and then subtract 17 from both sides to get $-3x^3 = -24$. Finally, we can divide both sides by -3 to get $x^3 = 8$. Since this isolates the cube of the variable, we can take the cube root of both sides to get $x = \sqrt[3]{8} = 2$.

One important but often overlooked point is that equations with an exponent greater than 1 may have more than one answer. The solution to $x^2 = 9$ isn't simply $x = 3$; it's $x = \pm 3$ (that is, $x = 3$ or $x = -3$). For a slightly more complicated example, consider the equation $(x - 1)^2 - 1 = 3$. Adding 1 to both sides yields $(x - 1)^2 = 4$; taking the square root of both sides yields $x - 1 = 2$. We can then add 1 to both sides to get $x = 3$. However, there's a second solution. We also have the possibility that $x - 1 = -2$, in which case $x = -1$. Both $x = 3$ and $x = -1$ are valid solutions, as can be verified by substituting them both into the original equation.

> **Review Video: Solving Equations with Exponents**
> Visit mometrix.com/academy and enter code: 514557
>
> **Review Video: Adding and Subtracting with Exponents**
> Visit mometrix.com/academy and enter code: 875756

Solving Equations with Absolute Values

When solving an equation with an absolute value, the first step is to isolate the absolute value term. We then consider two possibilities: when the expression inside the absolute value is positive or when it is negative. In the former case, the expression in the absolute value equals the expression on the other side of the equation; in the latter, it equals the additive inverse of that expression—the expression times negative one. We consider each case separately and finally check for spurious solutions.

For instance, consider solving $|2x - 1| + x = 5$ for x. We can first isolate the absolute value by moving the x to the other side: $|2x - 1| = -x + 5$. Now, we have two possibilities. First, that $2x - 1$ is positive, and hence $2x - 1 = -x + 5$. Rearranging and combining like terms yields $3x = 6$, and hence $x = 2$. The other possibility is that $2x - 1$ is negative, and hence $2x - 1 = -(-x + 5) = x - 5$. In this case, rearranging and combining like terms yields $x = -4$. Substituting $x = 2$ and $x = -4$ back into the original equation, we see that they are both valid solutions.

Note that the absolute value of a sum or difference applies to the sum or difference as a whole, not to the individual terms; in general, $|2x - 1|$ is not equal to $|2x + 1|$ or to $|2x| - 1$.

Review Video: Solving Absolute Value Equations
Visit mometrix.com/academy and enter code: 501208

Extraneous Solutions

An **extraneous solution** may arise when we square both sides of an equation (or raise both sides to an even power) as a step in solving it or under certain other operations on the equation. It is a solution to the squared or otherwise modified equation that is *not* a solution of the original equation. To identify an extraneous solution, it's useful when you solve an equation involving roots or absolute values to plug the solution back into the original equation to make sure it's valid.

Two-Variable Equations

Similar to methods for a one-variable equation, solving a two-variable equation involves isolating a variable: manipulating the equation so that a variable appears by itself on one side of the equation, and not at all on the other side. However, in a two-variable equation, you will usually only be able to isolate one of the variables; the other variable may appear on the other side along with constant terms, or with exponents or other functions. If an equation has multiple variables, the problem should tell you which variable to isolate.

Review Video: Solving Equations with Variables on Both Sides
Visit mometrix.com/academy and enter code: 402497

Graphing Equations

Graphical Solutions to Equations

When equations are shown graphically, they are usually shown on a **Cartesian coordinate plane**. The Cartesian coordinate plane consists of two number lines placed perpendicular to each other and intersecting at the zero point, also known as the origin. The horizontal number line is known as the x-axis, with positive values to the right of the origin, and negative values to the left of the origin. The vertical number line is known as the y-axis, with positive values above the origin, and negative values below the origin. Any point on the plane can be identified by an ordered pair in the form (x, y), called coordinates. The x-value of the coordinate is called the abscissa, and the y-value of the coordinate is called the ordinate. The two number lines divide the plane into **four quadrants**: I, II, III, and IV.

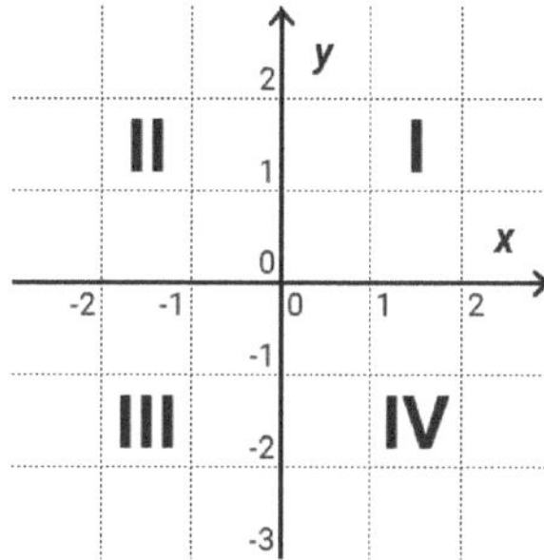

Note that in quadrant I $x > 0$ and $y > 0$, in quadrant II $x < 0$ and $y > 0$, in quadrant III $x < 0$ and $y < 0$, and in quadrant IV $x > 0$ and $y < 0$.

Recall that if the value of the slope of a line is positive, the line slopes upward from left to right. If the value of the slope is negative, the line slopes downward from left to right. If the y-coordinates are the same for two points on a line, the slope is 0 and the line is a **horizontal line**. If the x-coordinates are the same for two points on a line, there is no slope and the line is a **vertical line**. Two or more lines that have equivalent slopes are **parallel lines**. **Perpendicular lines** have slopes that are negative reciprocals of each other, such as $\frac{a}{b}$ and $\frac{-b}{a}$.

> **Review Video: Cartesian Coordinate Plane and Graphing**
> Visit mometrix.com/academy and enter code: 115173

Graphing Equations in Two Variables

One way of graphing an equation in two variables is to plot enough points to get an idea for its shape and then draw the appropriate curve through those points. A point can be plotted by substituting in a value for one variable and solving for the other. If the equation is linear, we only need two points and can then draw a straight line between them.

For example, consider the equation $y = 2x - 1$. This is a linear equation—both variables only appear raised to the first power—so we only need two points. When $x = 0$, $y = 2(0) - 1 = -1$. When $x = 2$, $y = 2(2) - 1 = 3$. We can therefore choose the points $(0, -1)$ and $(2, 3)$, and draw a line between them:

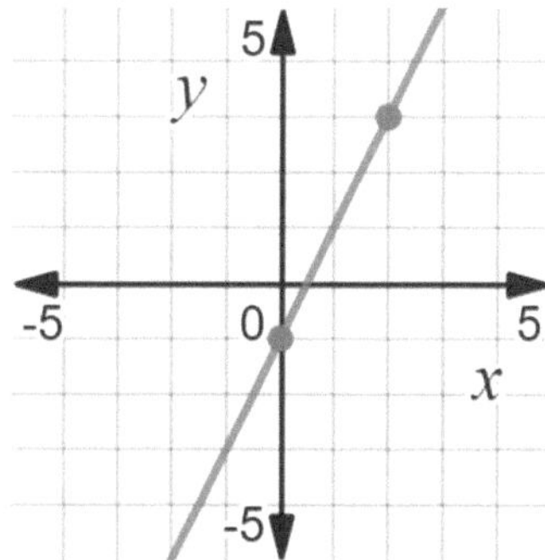

Inequalities

Commonly in algebra and other upper-level fields of math you find yourself working with mathematical expressions that do not equal each other. The statement comparing such expressions with symbols such as < (less than) or > (greater than) is called an *inequality*. An example of an inequality is $7x > 5$. To solve for x, simply divide both sides by 7 and the solution is shown to be $x > \frac{5}{7}$. Graphs of the solution set of inequalities are represented on a number line. Open circles are used to show that an expression approaches a number but is never quite equal to that number.

Review Video: Solving One-Step Inequalities
Visit mometrix.com/academy and enter code: 229684

Review Video: Solving Multi-Step Inequalities
Visit mometrix.com/academy and enter code: 347842

Review Video: Solving Inequalities Using All 4 Basic Operations
Visit mometrix.com/academy and enter code: 401111

TYPES OF INEQUALITIES

Conditional inequalities are those with certain values for the variable that will make the condition true and other values for the variable where the condition will be false. **Absolute inequalities** can have any real number as the value for the variable to make the condition true, while there is no real number value for the variable that will make the condition false. Solving inequalities is done by following the same rules for solving equations with the exception that when multiplying or dividing by a negative number the direction of the inequality sign must be flipped or reversed. **Double inequalities** are situations where two inequality statements apply to the same variable expression. Example: $-c < ax + b < c$.

Review Video: Conditional and Absolute Inequalities
Visit mometrix.com/academy and enter code: 980164

SOLVING INEQUALITIES

DETERMINING SOLUTIONS TO INEQUALITIES

To determine whether a coordinate is a solution of an inequality, you can substitute the values of the coordinate into the inequality, simplify, and check whether the resulting statement holds true. For instance, to determine whether $(-2,4)$ is a solution of the inequality $y \geq -2x + 3$, substitute the values into the inequality, $4 \geq -2(-2) + 3$. Simplify the right side of the inequality and the result is $4 \geq 7$, which is a false statement. Therefore, the coordinate is not a solution of the inequality. You can also use this method to determine which part of the graph of an inequality is shaded. The graph of $y \geq -2x + 3$ includes the solid line $y = -2x + 3$ and, since it excludes the point $(-2,4)$ to the left of the line, it is shaded to the right of the line.

Review Video: Graphing Linear Inequalities
Visit mometrix.com/academy and enter code: 439421

FLIPPING INEQUALITY SIGNS

When given an inequality, we can always turn the entire inequality around, swapping the two sides of the inequality and changing the inequality sign. For instance, $x + 2 > 2x - 3$ is equivalent to $2x - 3 < x + 2$. Aside from that, normally the inequality does not change if we carry out the same operation on both sides of the inequality. There is, however, one principal exception: if we *multiply* or *divide* both sides of the inequality by a *negative number*, the inequality is flipped. For example, if we take the inequality $-2x < 6$ and divide both sides by -2, the inequality flips and we are left with $x > -3$. This *only* applies to multiplication and division, and only with negative numbers.

Multiplying or dividing both sides by a positive number, or adding or subtracting any number regardless of sign, does not flip the inequality. Another special case that flips the inequality sign is when reciprocals are used. For instance, $3 > 2$ but the relation of the reciprocals is $\frac{1}{3} < \frac{1}{2}$.

COMPOUND INEQUALITIES

A **compound inequality** is an equality that consists of two inequalities combined with *and* or *or*. The two components of a proper compound inequality must be of opposite type: that is, one must be greater than (or greater than or equal to), the other less than (or less than or equal to). For instance, "$x + 1 < 2$ or $x + 1 > 3$" is a compound inequality, as is "$2x \geq 4$ and $2x \leq 6$." An *and* inequality can be written more compactly by having one inequality on each side of the common part: "$2x \geq 1$ and $2x \leq 6$," can also be written as $1 \leq 2x \leq 6$.

In order for the compound inequality to be meaningful, the two parts of an *and* inequality must overlap; otherwise, no numbers satisfy the inequality. On the other hand, if the two parts of an *or* inequality overlap, then *all* numbers satisfy the inequality and as such the inequality is usually not meaningful.

Solving a compound inequality requires solving each part separately. For example, given the compound inequality "$x + 1 < 2$ or $x + 1 > 3$," the first inequality, $x + 1 < 2$, reduces to $x < 1$, and the second part, $x + 1 > 3$, reduces to $x > 2$, so the whole compound inequality can be written as "$x < 1$ or $x > 2$." Similarly, $1 \leq 2x \leq 6$ can be solved by dividing each term by 2, yielding $\frac{1}{2} \leq x \leq 3$.

Review Video: Compound Inequalities
Visit mometrix.com/academy and enter code: 786318

SOLVING INEQUALITIES INVOLVING ABSOLUTE VALUES

To solve an inequality involving an absolute value, first isolate the term with the absolute value. Then proceed to treat the two cases separately as with an absolute value equation, but flipping the inequality in the case where the expression in the absolute value is negative (since that essentially involves multiplying both sides by −1.) The two cases are then combined into a compound inequality; if the absolute value is on the greater side of the inequality, then it is an *or* compound inequality, if on the lesser side, then it's an *and*.

Consider the inequality $2 + |x - 1| \geq 3$. We can isolate the absolute value term by subtracting 2 from both sides: $|x - 1| \geq 1$. Now, we're left with the two cases $x - 1 \geq 1$ or $x - 1 \leq -1$: note that in the latter, negative case, the inequality is flipped. $x - 1 \geq 1$ reduces to $x \geq 2$, and $x - 1 \leq -1$ reduces to $x \leq 0$. Since in the inequality $|x - 1| \geq 1$ the absolute value is on the greater side, the two cases combine into an *or* compound inequality, so the final, solved inequality is "$x \leq 0$ or $x \geq 2$."

Review Video: Solving Absolute Value Inequalities
Visit mometrix.com/academy and enter code: 997008

SOLVING INEQUALITIES INVOLVING SQUARE ROOTS

Solving an inequality with a square root involves two parts. First, we solve the inequality as if it were an equation, isolating the square root and then squaring both sides of the equation. Second, we restrict the solution to the set of values of x for which the value inside the square root sign is non-negative.

For example, in the inequality, $\sqrt{x-2}+1<5$, we can isolate the square root by subtracting 1 from both sides, yielding $\sqrt{x-2}<4$. Squaring both sides of the inequality yields $x-2<16$, so $x<18$. Since we can't take the square root of a negative number, we also require the part inside the square root to be non-negative. In this case, that means $x-2\geq 0$. Adding 2 to both sides of the inequality yields $x\geq 2$. Our final answer is a compound inequality combining the two simple inequalities: $x\geq 2$ and $x<18$, or $2\leq x<18$.

Note that we only get a compound inequality if the two simple inequalities are in opposite directions; otherwise, we take the one that is more restrictive.

The same technique can be used for other even roots, such as fourth roots. It is *not*, however, used for cube roots or other odd roots—negative numbers *do* have cube roots, so the condition that the quantity inside the root sign cannot be negative does not apply.

Review Video: Solving Inequalities Involving Square Roots
Visit mometrix.com/academy and enter code: 800288

SPECIAL CIRCUMSTANCES

Sometimes an inequality involving an absolute value or an even exponent is true for all values of x, and we don't need to do any further work to solve it. This is true if the inequality, once the absolute value or exponent term is isolated, says that term is greater than a negative number (or greater than or equal to zero). Since an absolute value or a number raised to an even exponent is *always* non-negative, this inequality is always true.

GRAPHING INEQUALITIES

GRAPHING SIMPLE INEQUALITIES

To graph a simple inequality, we first mark on the number line the value that signifies the end point of the inequality. If the inequality is strict (involves a less than or greater than), we use a hollow circle; if it is not strict (less than or equal to or greater than or equal to), we use a solid circle. We then fill in the part of the number line that satisfies the inequality: to the left of the marked point for less than (or less than or equal to), to the right for greater than (or greater than or equal to).

For example, we would graph the inequality $x<5$ by putting a hollow circle at 5 and filling in the part of the line to the left:

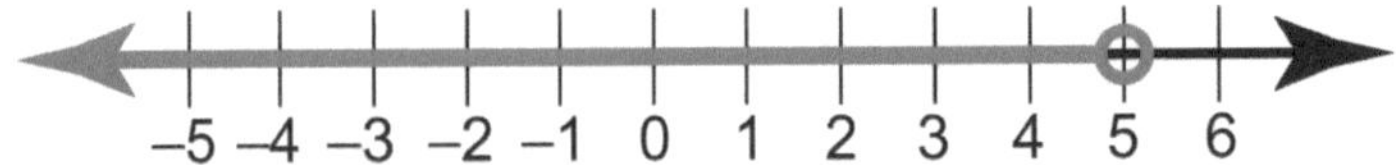

GRAPHING COMPOUND INEQUALITIES

To graph a compound inequality, we fill in both parts of the inequality for an *or* inequality, or the overlap between them for an *and* inequality. More specifically, we start by plotting the endpoints of each inequality on the number line. For an *or* inequality, we then fill in the appropriate side of the line for each inequality. Typically, the two component inequalities do not overlap, which means the shaded part is *outside* the two points. For an *and* inequality, we instead fill in the part of the line that meets both inequalities.

For the inequality "$x \leq -3$ or $x > 4$," we first put a solid circle at -3 and a hollow circle at 4. We then fill the parts of the line *outside* these circles:

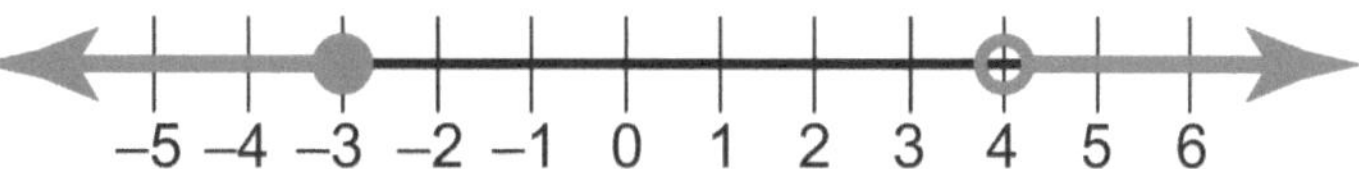

Graphing Inequalities Including Absolute Values

An inequality with an absolute value can be converted to a compound inequality. To graph the inequality, first convert it to a compound inequality, and then graph that normally. If the absolute value is on the greater side of the inequality, we end up with an *or* inequality; we plot the endpoints of the inequality on the number line and fill in the part of the line *outside* those points. If the absolute value is on the smaller side of the inequality, we end up with an *and* inequality; we plot the endpoints of the inequality on the number line and fill in the part of the line *between* those points.

For example, the inequality $|x + 1| \geq 4$ can be rewritten as $x \geq 3$ or $x \leq -5$. We place solid circles at the points 3 and -5 and fill in the part of the line *outside* them:

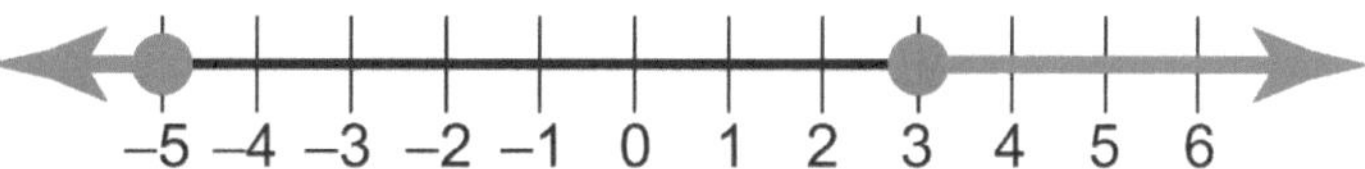

Graphing Inequalities in Two Variables

To graph an inequality in two variables, we first graph the border of the inequality. This means graphing the equation that we get if we replace the inequality sign with an equals sign. If the inequality is strict ($>$ or $<$), we graph the border with a dashed or dotted line; if it is not strict ($\geq$ or $\leq$), we use a solid line. We can then test any point not on the border to see if it satisfies the inequality. If it does, we shade in that side of the border; if not, we shade in the other side. As an example, consider $y > 2x + 2$. To graph this inequality, we first graph the border, $y = 2x + 2$. Since it is a strict inequality, we use a dashed line. Then, we choose a test point. This can be any point not on the border; in this case, we will choose the origin, (0,0). (This makes the calculation easy and is generally a good choice unless the border passes through the origin.) Putting this into the original inequality, we get $0 > 2(0) + 2$, i.e., $0 > 2$. This is *not* true, so we shade in the side of the border that does *not* include the point (0,0):

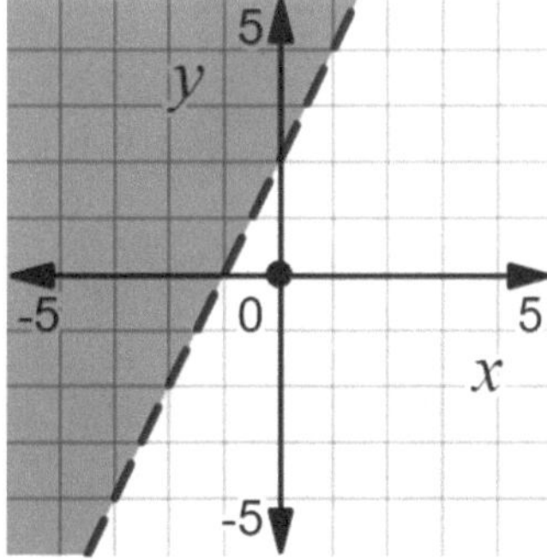

Graphing Compound Inequalities in Two Variables

One way to graph a compound inequality in two variables is to first graph each of the component inequalities. For an *and* inequality, we then shade in only the parts where the two graphs overlap; for an *or* inequality, we shade in any region that pertains to either of the individual inequalities.

Mathematics

Consider the graph of "$y \geq x - 1$ and $y \leq -x$":

We first shade in the individual inequalities:

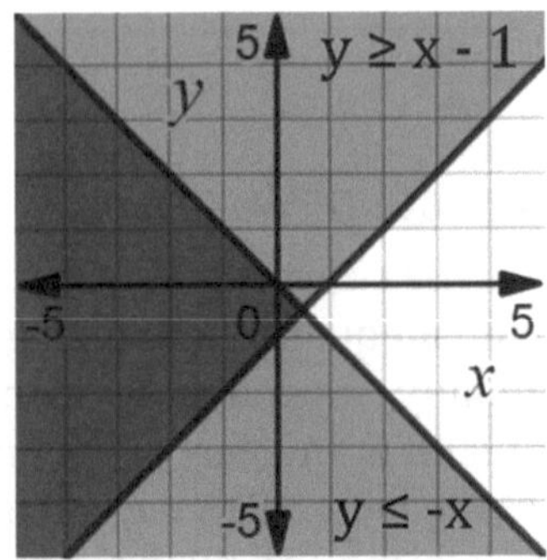

Now, since the compound inequality has an *and*, we only leave shaded the overlap—the part that pertains to *both* inequalities:

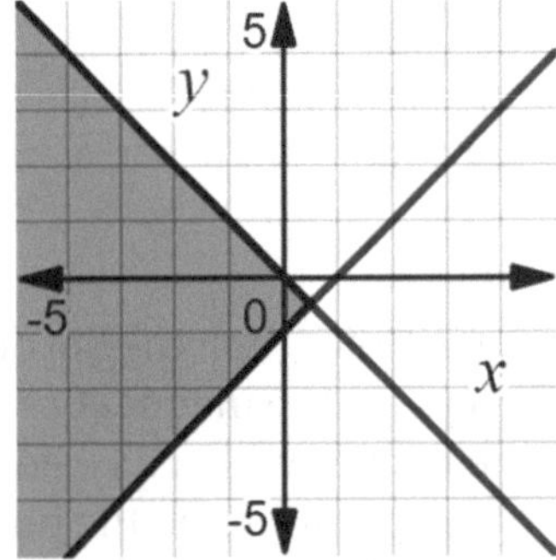

If instead the inequality had been "$y \geq x - 1$ or $y \leq -x$," our final graph would involve the *total* shaded area:

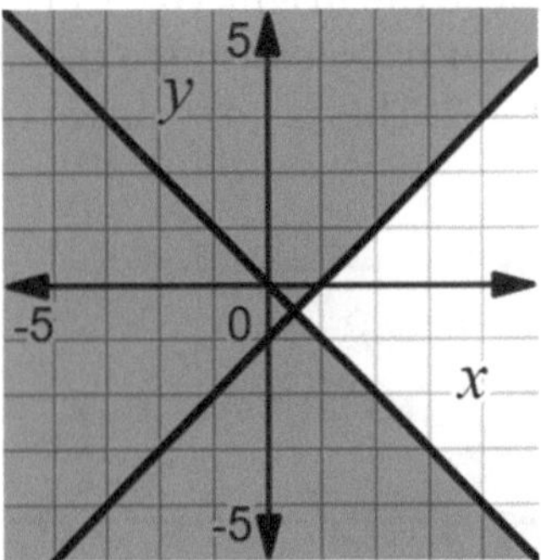

Review Video: Graphing Solutions to Inequalities
Visit mometrix.com/academy and enter code: 391281

Measurements and Time

Metric and Customary Measurements

Metric Measurement Prefixes

Giga-	One billion	1 *giga*watt is one billion watts
Mega-	One million	1 *mega*hertz is one million hertz
Kilo-	One thousand	1 *kilo*gram is one thousand grams
Deci-	One-tenth	1 *deci*meter is one-tenth of a meter
Centi-	One-hundredth	1 *centi*meter is one-hundredth of a meter
Milli-	One-thousandth	1 *milli*liter is one-thousandth of a liter
Micro-	One-millionth	1 *micro*gram is one-millionth of a gram

Review Video: How the Metric System Works
Visit mometrix.com/academy and enter code: 163709

Measurement Conversion

When converting between units, the goal is to maintain the same meaning but change the way it is displayed. In order to go from a larger unit to a smaller unit, multiply the number of the known amount by the equivalent amount. When going from a smaller unit to a larger unit, divide the number of the known amount by the equivalent amount.

For complicated conversions, it may be helpful to set up conversion fractions. In these fractions, one fraction is the **conversion factor**. The other fraction has the unknown amount in the numerator. So, the known value is placed in the denominator. Sometimes, the second fraction has the known value from the problem in the numerator and the unknown in the denominator. Multiply the two fractions to get the converted measurement. Note that since the numerator and the denominator of the factor are equivalent, the value of the fraction is 1. That is why we can say that the result in the new units is equal to the result in the old units even though they have different numbers.

It can often be necessary to chain known conversion factors together. As an example, consider converting 512 square inches to square meters. We know that there are 2.54 centimeters in an inch and 100 centimeters in a meter, and we know we will need to square each of these factors to achieve the conversion we are looking for.

$$\frac{512\text{ in}^2}{1} \times \left(\frac{2.54\text{ cm}}{1\text{ in}}\right)^2 \times \left(\frac{1\text{ m}}{100\text{ cm}}\right)^2 = \frac{512\ \cancel{\text{in}^2}}{1} \times \left(\frac{6.4516\ \cancel{\text{cm}^2}}{1\ \cancel{\text{in}^2}}\right) \times \left(\frac{1\text{ m}^2}{10{,}000\ \cancel{\text{cm}^2}}\right) = 0.330\text{ m}^2$$

Review Video: Measurement Conversions
Visit mometrix.com/academy and enter code: 316703

Review Video: Converting Kilograms to Pounds
Visit mometrix.com/academy and enter code: 241463

Common Units and Equivalents

Metric Equivalents

1000 μg (microgram)	1 mg
1000 mg (milligram)	1 g
1000 g (gram)	1 kg
1000 kg (kilogram)	1 metric ton
1000 mL (milliliter)	1 L
1000 μm (micrometer)	1 mm
1000 mm (millimeter)	1 m
100 cm (centimeter)	1 m
1000 m (meter)	1 km

Distance and Area Measurement

Unit	Abbreviation	US equivalent	Metric equivalent
Inch	in	1 inch	2.54 centimeters
Foot	ft	12 inches	0.305 meters
Yard	yd	3 feet	0.914 meters
Mile	mi	5280 feet	1.609 kilometers
Acre	ac	4840 square yards	0.405 hectares
Square Mile	sq. mi. or $mi.^2$	640 acres	2.590 square kilometers

Capacity Measurements

Unit	Abbreviation	US equivalent	Metric equivalent
Fluid Ounce	fl oz	8 fluid drams	29.573 milliliters
Cup	c	8 fluid ounces	0.237 liter
Pint	pt.	16 fluid ounces	0.473 liter
Quart	qt.	2 pints	0.946 liter
Gallon	gal.	4 quarts	3.785 liters
Teaspoon	t or tsp.	1 fluid dram	5 milliliters
Tablespoon	T or tbsp.	4 fluid drams	15 or 16 milliliters
Cubic Centimeter	cc or cm^3	0.271 drams	1 milliliter

Weight Measurements

Unit	Abbreviation	US equivalent	Metric equivalent
Ounce	oz	16 drams	28.35 grams
Pound	lb	16 ounces	453.6 grams
Ton	tn.	2,000 pounds	907.2 kilograms

Volume and Weight Measurement Clarifications

Always be careful when using ounces and fluid ounces. They are not equivalent.

1 pint = 16 fluid ounces	1 fluid ounce $\neq$ 1 ounce
1 pound = 16 ounces	1 pint $\neq$ 1 pound

Having one pint of something does not mean you have one pound of it. In the same way, just because something weighs one pound does not mean that its volume is one pint.

In the United States, the word "ton" by itself refers to a short ton or a net ton. Do not confuse this with a long ton (also called a gross ton) or a metric ton (also spelled *tonne*), which have different measurement equivalents.

$$1 \text{ US ton} = 2000 \text{ pounds} \qquad \neq \qquad 1 \text{ metric ton} = 1000 \text{ kilograms}$$

Military Time

The **24-hour clock** is a time system used by the military and on some digital clocks. On the 24-hour clock, minutes and seconds are the same as the standard 12-hour clock. However, time is expressed in 4 figures, and the hours run from 0000 hour (12 a.m.) to 2359 hours (11:59 p.m.).

To convert from 12-hour to 24-hour time, remove the colon and:

- for a.m. times, if the time has 3 digits, add a 0 to the beginning (e.g., 8:12 a.m. becomes 0812 hours). For times between 12 a.m. and 1 a. m., replace the 12 with a pair of zeros (e.g., 12:41 a.m. becomes 0041 hours).
- for p.m. times, add 12 to the hour number (e.g., 3:40 p.m. = 1540 hours), except for times between 12 p.m. and 1 p.m., which do not require any further change.

To convert from 24-hour to 12-hour time, add a colon between the second and third digits. If the first two digits are less than 12, the time is a.m.; otherwise it is p.m. If the first two digits are zeros, the hour becomes 12 a.m. (e.g., 0020 becomes 12:20 a.m.) If only the first digit is zero, remove it (e.g., 0730 becomes 7:30 a.m.). If the first two digits are greater than 12, subtract 12 (e.g., 2325 becomes 11:25 p.m.).

Science

Transform passive reading into active learning! After immersing yourself in this chapter, put your comprehension to the test by taking a quiz. The insights you gained will stay with you longer this way. Scan the QR code to go directly to the chapter quiz interface for this study guide. If you're using a computer, simply visit the bonus page at **mometrix.com/bonus948/kaplannursing** and click the Chapter Quizzes link.

Scientific Inquiry and Reasoning

Scientific Inquiry

The concept of **scientific inquiry** refers to the idea of how one thinks and asks questions in a logical way to gain trustworthy information. The underlying motivation of science is to try to understand the natural world. Much of human thought is based on assumptions about how things work that may or may not be true. The goal of scientific inquiry is to test those assumptions to gain a greater understanding of the world with good questions and objective tests, and then re-use what was learned to ask better questions. The more we understand about the natural world, the better the questions we can ask, and that is the general idea behind scientific inquiry. The applied practice of scientific inquiry is to ask questions in a systematic method, called the scientific method.

Scientific Knowledge

Scientific knowledge refers to any topic that is studied **empirically**, meaning that it is based on observation of a **phenomenon** in an objective way. The body of **scientific knowledge** is often broken down into several domains including biology, ecology, Earth science, space science, physics, and chemistry. These each have further subdomains and are overlapping in many ways. For instance, ecology is the study of ecosystems, which are made up of biological factors and geological factors, so it contains elements of both biology and Earth science. Each of these domains is subject to the concepts of scientific inquiry, such as the scientific method, scientific facts, hypotheses, and scientific laws.

Important Terminology

- A **phenomenon** is an event or effect that is observed.
- A **scientific fact** is considered an objective and verifiable observation. Usually, a fact can be repeated or demonstrated to others.
- A **scientific theory** is a proposition explaining why or how something happens and is built on scientific facts and laws. Scientific theories can be tested, but are not fully proven. If new evidence is found that disproves the theory, it is no longer considered true.
- A **hypothesis** is an educated guess that is not yet proven. It is used to predict the outcome of an experiment in an attempt to solve a problem or answer a question.
- A **law** is an explanation of events that always leads to the same outcome. It is a fact that an object falls. The law of gravity explains why an object falls. The theory of relativity, although generally accepted, has been neither proven nor disproved.
- A **model** is used to explain something on a smaller scale or in simpler terms to provide an example. It is a representation of an idea that can be used to explain events or applied to new situations to predict outcomes or determine results.

History of Scientific Knowledge

When one examines the history of **scientific knowledge**, it is clear that it is constantly **evolving**. The body of facts, models, theories, and laws grows and changes over time. In other words, one scientific discovery leads to the next. Some advances in science and technology have important and long-lasting effects on science and society. Some discoveries were so alien to the accepted beliefs of the time that not only were they rejected as wrong, but were also considered outright blasphemy. Today, however, many beliefs once considered incorrect have become an ingrained part of scientific knowledge, and have also been the basis of new advances. Examples of advances include: Copernicus's heliocentric view of the universe, Newton's laws of motion and planetary orbits, relativity, geologic time scale, plate tectonics, atomic theory, nuclear physics, biological evolution, germ theory, industrial revolution, molecular biology, information and communication, quantum theory, galactic universe, and medical and health technology.

Scientific Inquiry and Scientific Method

Scientists use a number of generally accepted techniques collectively known as the **scientific method**. The scientific method generally involves carrying out the following steps:

- Identifying a problem or posing a question
- Formulating a hypothesis or an educated guess
- Conducting experiments or tests that will provide a basis to solve the problem or answer the question
- Observing the results of the test
- Drawing conclusions

An important part of the scientific method is using acceptable experimental techniques. Objectivity is also important if valid results are to be obtained. Another important part of the scientific method is peer review. It is essential that experiments be performed and data be recorded in such a way that experiments can be reproduced to verify results. Historically, the scientific method has been taught with a more linear approach, but it is important to recognize that the scientific method should be a cyclical or **recursive process**. This means that as hypotheses are tested and more is learned, the questions should continue to change to reflect the changing body of knowledge. One cycle of experimentation is not enough.

Review Video: The Scientific Method
Visit mometrix.com/academy and enter code: 191386

Metric and International System of Units

The **metric system** is the accepted standard of measurement in the scientific community. The **International System of Units (SI)** is a set of measurements (including the metric system) that is almost globally accepted. The United States, Liberia, and Myanmar have not accepted this system. **Standardization** is important because it allows the results of experiments to be compared and reproduced without the need to laboriously convert measurements. The SI is based partially on the **meter-kilogram-second (MKS) system** rather than the **centimeter-gram-second (CGS) system**. The MKS system considers meters, kilograms, and seconds to be the basic units of measurement, while the CGS system considers centimeters, grams, and seconds to be the basic units of measurement. Under the MKS system, the length of an object would be expressed as 1 meter instead of 100 centimeters, which is how it would be described under the CGS system.

Review Video: Metric System Conversions
Visit mometrix.com/academy and enter code: 163709

Basic Units of Measurement

Using the **metric system** is generally accepted as the preferred method for taking measurements. Having a **universal standard** allows individuals to interpret measurements more easily, regardless of where they are located. The basic units of measurement are: the **meter**, which measures length; the **liter**, which measures volume; and the **gram**, which measures mass. The metric system starts with a base unit and increases or decreases in units of 10. The prefix and the base unit combined are used to indicate an amount. For example, deka- is 10 times the base unit. A dekameter is 10 meters; a dekaliter is 10 liters; and a dekagram is 10 grams. The prefix hecto- refers to 100 times the base amount; kilo- is 1,000 times the base amount. The prefixes that indicate a fraction of the base unit are deci-, which is $\frac{1}{10}$ of the base unit; centi-, which is $\frac{1}{100}$ of the base unit; and milli-, which is $\frac{1}{1,000}$ of the base unit.

Common Prefixes

The prefixes for multiples are as follows:

Deka	(da)	$\mathbf{10^1}$ (deka is the American spelling, but deca is also used)
Hecto	(h)	10^2
Kilo	(k)	10^3
Mega	(M)	10^6
Giga	(G)	10^9
Tera	(T)	10^{12}

The prefixes for subdivisions are as follows:

Deci	(d)	$\mathbf{10^{-1}}$
Centi	(c)	10^{-2}
Milli	(m)	10^{-3}
Micro	(μ)	10^{-6}
Nano	(n)	10^{-9}
Pico	(p)	10^{-12}

The rule of thumb is that prefixes greater than 10^3 are capitalized when abbreviating. Abbreviations do not need a period after them. A decimeter (dm) is a tenth of a meter, a deciliter (dL) is a tenth of a liter, and a decigram (dg) is a tenth of a gram. Pluralization is understood. For example, when referring to 5 mL of water, no "s" needs to be added to the abbreviation.

Basic SI Units of Measurement

SI uses **second(s)** to measure time. Fractions of seconds are usually measured in metric terms using prefixes such as millisecond ($\frac{1}{1,000}$ of a second) or nanosecond ($\frac{1}{1,000,000,000}$ of a second). Increments of time larger than a second are measured in **minutes** and **hours**, which are multiples of 60 and 24. An example of this is a swimmer's time in the 800-meter freestyle being described as 7:32.67, meaning 7 minutes, 32 seconds, and 67 one-hundredths of a second. One second is equal to $\frac{1}{60}$ of a minute, $\frac{1}{3,600}$ of an hour, and $\frac{1}{86,400}$ of a day. Other SI base units are the **ampere** (A) (used to measure electric current), the **kelvin** (K) (used to measure thermodynamic temperature), the **candela** (cd) (used to measure luminous intensity), and the **mole** (mol) (used to measure the amount of a substance at a molecular level). **Meter** (m) is used to measure length and **kilogram** (kg) is used to measure mass.

Significant Figures

The mathematical concept of **significant figures** or **significant digits** is often used to determine the accuracy of measurements or the level of confidence one has in a specific measurement. The significant figures of a measurement include all the digits known with certainty plus one estimated or uncertain digit. There are a number of rules for determining which digits are considered "important" or "interesting." They are: all non-zero digits are *significant*, zeros between digits are *significant*, and leading and trailing zeros are *not significant* unless they appear to the right of the non-zero digits in a decimal. For example, in 0.01230 the significant digits are 1230, and this number would be said to be accurate to the hundred-thousandths place. The zero indicates that the amount has actually been measured as 0. Other zeros are considered place holders, and are not important. A decimal point may be placed after zeros to indicate their importance (in 100. for example). **Estimating**, on the other hand, involves approximating a value rather than calculating the exact number. This may be used to quickly determine a value that is close to the actual number when complete accuracy does not matter or is not possible. In science, estimation may be used when it is impossible to measure or calculate an exact amount, or to quickly approximate an answer when true calculations would be time consuming.

Graphs and Charts

Graphs and charts are effective ways to present scientific data such as observations, statistical analyses, and comparisons between dependent variables and independent variables. On a line chart, the **independent variable** (the one that is being manipulated for the experiment) is represented on the horizontal axis (the x-axis). Any **dependent variables** (the ones that may change as the independent variable changes) are represented on the y-axis. An **XY** or **scatter plot** is often used to plot many points. A "best fit" line is drawn, which allows outliers to be identified more easily. Charts and their axes should have titles. The x and y interval units should be evenly spaced and labeled. Other types of charts are **bar charts** and **histograms**, which can be used to compare differences between the data collected for two variables. A **pie chart** can graphically show the relation of parts to a whole.

Review Video: Identifying Variables
Visit mometrix.com/academy and enter code: 627181

Review Video: Data Interpretation of Graphs
Visit mometrix.com/academy and enter code: 200439

Data Presentation

Data collected during a science lab can be organized and **presented** in any number of ways. While **straight narrative** is a suitable method for presenting some lab results, it is not a suitable way to present numbers and quantitative measurements. These types of observations can often be better presented with **tables** and **graphs**. Data that is presented in tables and organized in rows and columns may also be used to make graphs quite easily. Other methods of presenting data include illustrations, photographs, video, and even audio formats. In a **formal report**, tables and figures are labeled and referred to by their labels. For example, a picture of a bubbly solution might be labeled Figure 1, Bubbly Solution. It would be referred to in the text in the following way: "The reaction created bubbles 10 mm in size, as shown in Figure 1, Bubbly Solution." Graphs are also labeled as figures. Tables are labeled in a different way. Examples include: Table 1, Results of Statistical Analysis, or Table 2, Data from Lab 2.

Statistical Precision and Errors

Errors that occur during an experiment can be classified into two categories: random errors and systematic errors. **Random errors** can result in collected data that is wildly different from the rest of the data, or they may result in data that is indistinguishable from the rest. Random errors are not consistent across the data set. In large data sets, random errors may contribute to the variability of data, but they will not affect the average. Random errors are sometimes referred to as noise. They may be caused by a student's inability to take the same measurement in exactly the same way or by outside factors that are not considered variables, but influence the data. A **systematic error** will show up consistently across a sample or data set, and may be the result of a flaw in the experimental design. This type of error affects the average, and is also known as bias.

Scientific Notation

Scientific notation is used because values in science can be very large or very small, which makes them unwieldy. A number in **decimal notation** is 93,000,000. In **scientific notation**, it is 9.3×10^7. The first number, 9.3, is the **coefficient**. It is always greater than or equal to 1 and less than 10. This number is followed by a multiplication sign. The base is always 10 in scientific notation. If the number is greater than ten, the exponent is positive. If the number is between zero and one, the exponent is negative. The first digit of the number is followed by a decimal point and then the rest of the number. In this case, the number is 9.3, and the decimal point was moved seven places to the right from the end of the number to get 93,000,000. The number of places moved, seven, is the exponent.

Statistical Terminology

- **Mean** - The average, found by taking the sum of a set of numbers and dividing by the number of numbers in the set.
- **Median** - The middle number in a set of numbers sorted from least to greatest. If the set has an even number of entries, the median is the average of the two in the middle.
- **Mode** - The value that appears most frequently in a data set. There may be more than one mode. If no value appears more than once, there is no mode.
- **Range** - The difference between the highest and lowest numbers in a data set.
- **Standard deviation** - Measures the dispersion of a data set or how far from the mean a single data point is likely to be.
- **Regression analysis** - A method of analyzing sets of data and sets of variables that involves studying how the typical value of the dependent variable changes when any one of the independent variables is varied and the other independent variables remain fixed.

Review Video: Mean, Median, and Mode
Visit mometrix.com/academy and enter code: 286207

Review Video: Standard Deviation
Visit mometrix.com/academy and enter code: 419469

Chemical Structures and Properties of Biologically Important Molecules

Chemical Bonding Properties of Carbon

Carbon is considered to be the central atom of organic compounds. Carbon atoms each have four valence electrons and require four more electrons to have a stable outer shell. Due to the repulsion between the valence electrons, the bond sites are all equidistant from each other. This enables carbon to form longs chains and rings. Carbon atoms can form four single covalent bonds with other atoms. For example, methane (CH_4) consists of one carbon atom singly bonded to four separate hydrogen atoms. Carbon atoms can also form double or triple covalent bonds. For example, an oxygen atom can form a double bond with a carbon atom, and a nitrogen atom can form a triple bond with a carbon atom.

Organic and Inorganic Molecules

Organic molecules contain carbon and hydrogen. Because carbon can form four covalent bonds, organic molecules can be very complex structures. Organic molecules can have carbon backbones that form long chains, branched chains, or even rings. Organic compounds tend to be less soluble in water than inorganic compounds. Organic compounds are often classified as either natural (found in plants and animals) or as synthetic (made via laboratory or industrial processes). **Inorganic molecules** generally do not contain carbon-carbon or carbon-hydrogen bonds, but there are some exceptions. Inorganic compounds include salts and metals. Specific examples of inorganic molecules include sodium chloride, oxygen, and carbon dioxide.

Covalent Bonds

Chemical bonds are the attractive forces that bind atoms together to form molecules. Chemical bonds include covalent bonds, ionic bonds, and metallic bonds. **Covalent bonds** are formed from the sharing of electron pairs between two atoms in a molecule. In organic molecules, carbon atoms form single, double, or triple covalent bonds. Organic compounds including proteins, carbohydrates, lipids, and nucleic acids are molecular compounds formed by covalent bonds.

Review Video: Covalent Bonds
Visit mometrix.com/academy and enter code: 482899

Hydrogen Bonds

Intermolecular forces are the attractive forces between molecules. Intermolecular forces include hydrogen bonds, London or dispersion forces, and dipole-dipole forces. **Hydrogen bonds** are the attractive forces between molecules containing hydrogen atoms covalently bonded to oxygen, fluorine, or nitrogen. Hydrogen bonds bind the two strands of a DNA molecule to each other. Two hydrogen bonds join each adenosine and thymine, and three hydrogen bonds join each cytosine and guanine.

ATP

Adenosine triphosphate (ATP) is the energy source for most cellular functions. Each ATP molecule is a nucleotide consisting of a central ribose sugar flanked by a purine base and a chain of three phosphate groups. The purine base is adenine, and when adenine is joined to ribose, an adenosine is formed, explaining the name adenosine triphosphate. If one phosphate is removed from the end of the molecule, adenosine diphosphate (ADP) is formed.

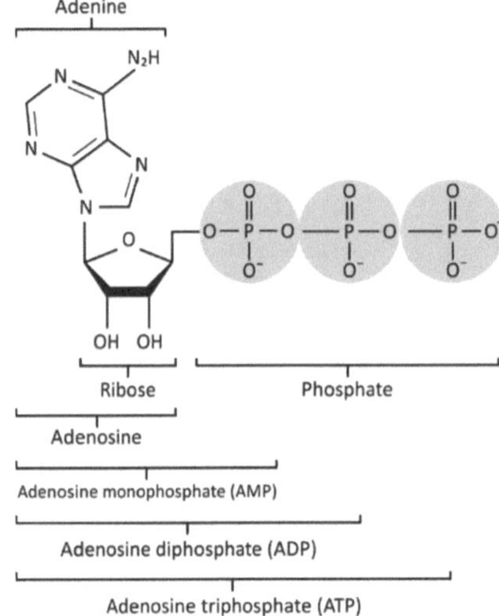

Properties of Water

Water exhibits numerous properties. Water has a high surface tension due to the cohesion between water molecules from the hydrogen bonds between the molecules. The capillary action of water is also due to this cohesion, and the adhesion of water is due to its polarity. Water is an excellent solvent due to its polarity and is considered the universal solvent. Water exists naturally as a solid, liquid, and gas. The density of water decreases as ice freezes and forms crystals in the solid phase. Water is most dense at 4 °C. Water can act as an acid or base in chemical reactions. Pure water is an insulator because it has virtually no ions. Water has a high specific heat capacity due to its low molecular mass and bent molecular shape.

> **Review Video: Properties of Water**
> Visit mometrix.com/academy and enter code: 279526

Biological Macromolecules

Macromolecules are large molecules made up of smaller organic molecules. Four classes of macromolecules include carbohydrates, nucleic acids, proteins, and lipids. Carbohydrates, proteins, and nucleic acids are polymers that are formed when the monomers are joined together in a dehydration process. In this dehydration process, the monomers are joined by a covalent bond and a water molecule is released. The monomers in carbohydrates are simple sugars such as glucose, while polysaccharides are polymers of carbohydrates. The monomers in proteins are amino acids. The amino acids form polypeptide chains, which are folded into proteins. The monomers in nucleic acids are nucleotides. Lipids are not actually considered to be polymers. Lipids typically are classified as fats, phospholipids, or steroids.

> **Review Video: Macromolecules**
> Visit mometrix.com/academy and enter code: 220156

Biological Processes Dependent on Chemical Principles

Biochemical Pathways

Autotrophs that use light to produce energy use **photosynthesis** as a biochemical pathway. In eukaryotic autotrophs photosynthesis takes place in chloroplasts. Prokaryotic autotrophs that use inorganic chemical reactions to produce energy use **chemosynthesis** as a biochemical pathway. Heterotrophs require food and use **cellular respiration** to release energy from chemical bonds in the food. All organisms use cellular respiration to release energy from stored food. Cellular respiration can be aerobic or anaerobic. Most eukaryotes use cellular respiration that takes place in the mitochondria.

Photosynthesis

Photosynthesis is a food-making process that occurs in three processes: light-capturing events, light-dependent reactions, and light-independent reactions. In light-capturing events, the thylakoids of the chloroplasts, which contain chlorophyll and accessory pigments, absorb light energy and produce excited electrons. Thylakoids also contain enzymes and electron-transport molecules. Molecules involved in this process are arranged in groups called photosystems. In light-dependent reactions, the excited electrons from the light-capturing events are moved by electron transport in a series of steps in which they are used to split water into hydrogen and oxygen ions. The oxygen is released, and the $NADP^+$ bonds with the hydrogen atoms and forms NADPH. ATP is produced from the excited elections. The light-independent reactions use this ATP, NADPH, and carbon dioxide to produce sugars.

> **Review Video: Photosynthesis**
> Visit mometrix.com/academy and enter code: 227035

C_3 and C_4 Photosynthesis

Plants undergo an additional process during photosynthesis that is known as photorespiration. Photorespiration is a wasteful process that uses energy and decreases sugar synthesis. This process occurs when the enzyme rubisco binds to oxygen rather than atmospheric carbon dioxide. There are three different processes that plants use to fix carbon during photosynthesis and these include C_3, C_4, and crassulacean acid metabolism (CAM). Some plants, such as C_4 and CAM plants, can decrease photorespiration and therefore minimize energy lost while C_3 plants, which make up more than 85% of plants, have no special adaptations to stop photorespiration from occuring. C_3 and C_4 plants are named for the type of carbon molecule (three-carbon or four-carbon) that is made during the first step of the reaction. The first step of the C_3 process involves the formation of two three-carbon molecules (3-phosphoglycerate; 3-PGA) from carbon dioxide being fixed by the enzyme. The first step of C_4 photosynthesis is carbon dioxide beign fixed by the enzyme PEP carboxylase, which unlike rubisco does not have the ability to bind to oxygen. This fixation forms a four-carbon molecule (oxaloaceate) and these initial steps occur in the mesophyll cell. Next, oxaloacetate is converted into a malate, a molecule that can enter the bundle sheath cells, and then is broken down to release carbon dioxide. From there, the carbon dioxide is fixed by rubisco as it undergoes the Calvin cycle seen in C_3 photosynthesis. Because C_4 plants undergo an initial step that allows carbon dioxide to be more readily available, with the use of malate, photorespiration is minimized.

Crassulacean Acid Metabolism

Crassulacean acid metabolism (CAM) is a form of photosynthesis adapted to dry environments. While C_4 plants separate the Calvin cycle via space, or by having different cells for different functions and processes, CAM plants separate the processes by time of day. During the night, pores of the plant leaves, called stomata, open to receive carbon dioxide, which combines with PEP carboxylase to form oxaloacetate. Oxaloacetate is eventually converted into malate, which is stored in vacuoles until the next day. During the following day, the stomata are closed and the malate is transported to chloroplasts, where malate is broken down into pyruvate (three-carbon molecule) and carbon dioxide. The carbon dioxide released from malate is used in photosynthesis during the daytime. One advantage of the CAM cycle is that it minimizes loss of water through the stomata during the daytime. A second advantage is that concentrating carbon dioxide in the chloroplasts in this manner increases the efficiency of the enzyme rubisco to fix carbon dioxide and complete the Calvin cycle.

AEROBIC RESPIRATION

Aerobic cellular respiration is a series of enzyme-controlled chemical reactions in which oxygen reacts with glucose to produce carbon dioxide and water, releasing energy in the form of adenosine triphosphate (ATP). Cellular respiration occurs in a series of three processes: glycolysis, the Krebs cycle, and the electron-transport system.

Review Video: Aerobic Respiration
Visit mometrix.com/academy and enter code: 770290

GLYCOLYSIS

Glycolysis is a series of enzyme-controlled chemical reactions that occur in the cell's cytoplasm. Each glucose molecule is split in half to produce two pyruvic acid molecules, four ATP molecules, and two NADH molecules. Because two ATP molecules are used to split the glucose molecule, the net ATP yield for glycolysis is two ATP molecules.

Review Video: Glycolysis
Visit mometrix.com/academy and enter code: 466815

KREBS CYCLE

The **Krebs cycle** is also called the citric acid cycle or the tricarboxylic acid cycle (TCA). It is a **catabolic pathway** in which the bonds of glucose and occasionally fats or lipids are broken down and reformed into ATP. It is a respiration process that uses oxygen and produces carbon dioxide, water, and ATP. Cells require energy from ATP to synthesize proteins from amino acids and replicate DNA. The cycle is acetyl CoA, citric acid, isocitric acid, ketoglutaric acid (products are amino acids and CO_2), succinyl CoA, succinic acid, fumaric acid, malic acid, and oxaloacetic acid. One of the products of the Krebs cycle is NADH, which is then used in the electron chain transport system to manufacture ATP. From glycolysis, pyruvate is oxidized in a step linking to the Krebs cycle. After the Krebs cycle, NADH and succinate are oxidized in the electron transport chain.

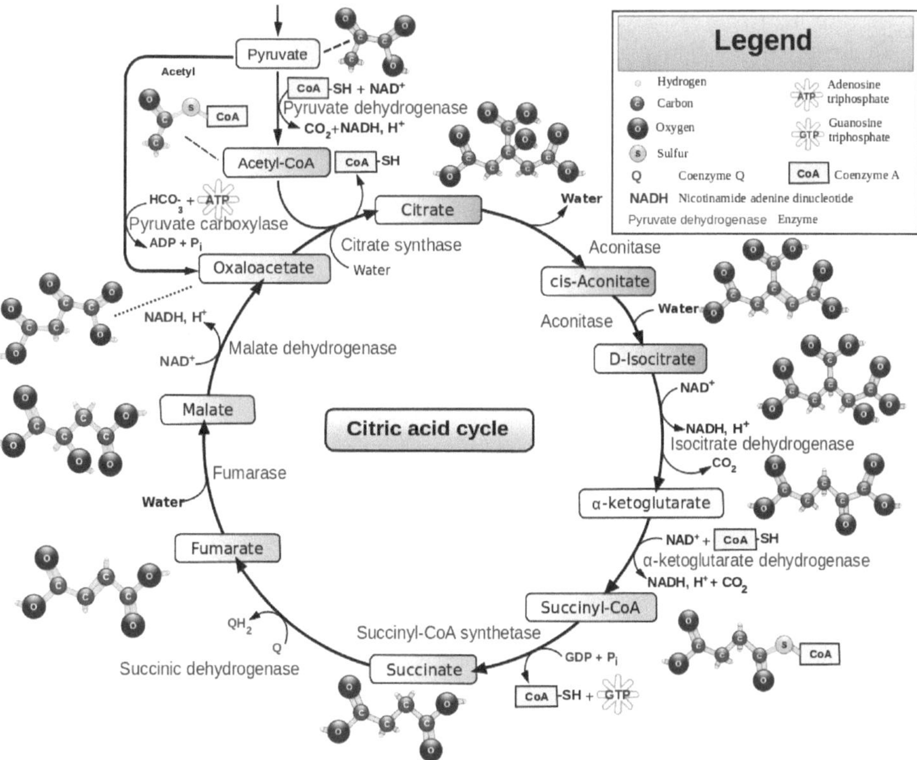

ELECTRON TRANSPORT CHAIN

The **electron transport chain** is part of phosphorylation, whereby electrons are transported from enzyme to enzyme until they reach a final acceptor. The electron transport chain includes a series of oxidizing and reducing molecules involved in the release of energy. In **redox reactions**, electrons are removed from a substrate (oxidative) and H^+ (protons) can also be simultaneously removed. A substrate gains electrons during reduction. For example, when glucose is oxidized, electrons are lost and energy is released. There are enzymes in the membranes of mitochondria. The electrons are carried from one enzyme to another by a co-enzyme. Protons are also released to the other side of the membrane. For example, FAD and $FADH_2$ are used in oxidative phosphorylation. FAD is reduced to $FADH_2$. Electrons are stored there and then sent onward, and the $FADH_2$ becomes FAD again. In aerobic respiration, the final electron acceptor is O_2. In anaerobic respiration, it is something other than O_2.

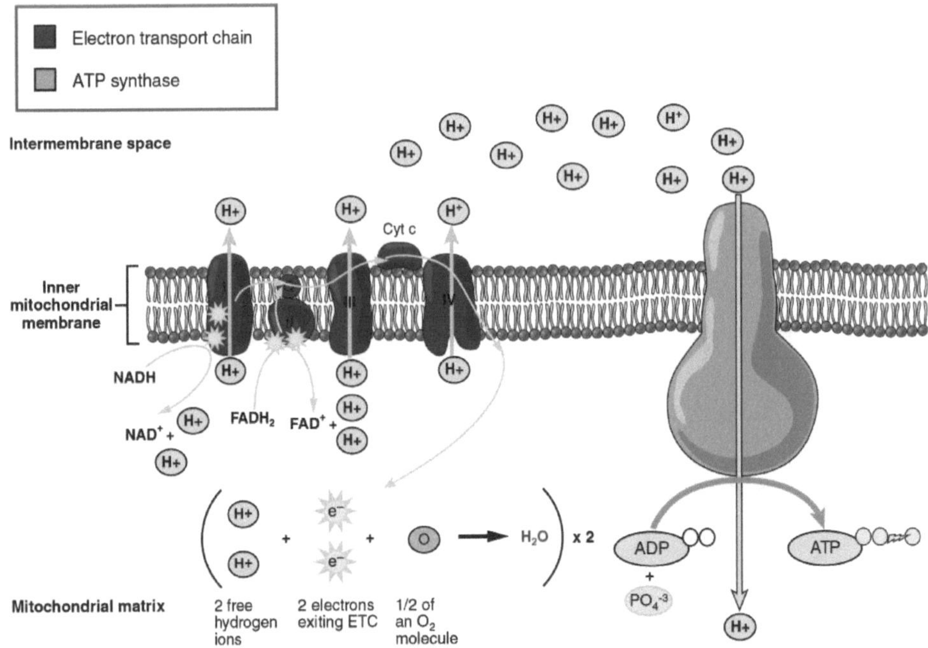

Fermentation

Fermentation is an anaerobic reaction in which glucose is only partially broken down. It releases energy through the oxidation of sugars or other types of organic molecules. Oxygen is sometimes involved, but not always. It is different from respiration in that it uses neither the Krebs cycle nor the electron transport chain and the final electron acceptor is an organic molecule. It uses **substrate-level phosphorylation** to form ATP. NAD^+ is reduced to NADH and NADH further reduces pyruvic acid to various end products. Fermentation can lead to excess waste products and is less efficient than aerobic respiration. **Homolactic fermentation** refers to lactic acid fermentation in which the sugars are converted to lactic acid only (there is one end product). In **heterolactic fermentation**, the sugars are converted to a range of products.

Examples of Fermentation

Lactic acid fermentation is the breakdown of glucose and six-carbon sugars into lactic acid to release energy. It is an anaerobic process, meaning that it does not require oxygen. It can occur in muscle cells and is also performed by streptococcus and lactobacillus bacteria. It can also be used to making yogurt and other food products.

Alcohol fermentation is the breakdown of glucose and six-carbon sugars into ethanol and carbon dioxide to release energy. It is an anaerobic process. It is performed by yeast and used in the production of alcoholic beverages.

Chemosynthesis

Chemosynthesis is the food-making process of chemoautotrophs in extreme environments such as deep-sea-vents, or hydrothermal vents. Unlike photosynthesis, chemosynthesis does not require light. In general, chemosynthesis involves the oxidation of inorganic substances to make a sugar, but there are several species that use different pathways or processses. For example, sulfur bacteria live near or in deep-sea vents and oxidize hydrogen sulfide released from those vents to make a sugar. Instead of sunlight, chemosynthesis uses the energy stored in the chemical bonds of chemicals such as hydrogen sulfide to produce food. During chemosynthesis, the electrons that are removed from the inorganic molecules are combined with carbon dioxide and oxygen to produce sugar, sulfur, and water. Some bacteria use metal ions such as iron and magnesium to obtain the needed electrons. For example, methanobacteria such as those found in human intestines combine carbon dioxide and hydrogen gas and release methane as a waste product. Nitrogen bacteria such as nitrogen-fixing bacteria in the nodules of legumes convert atmospheric nitrogen into nitrates.

Differences Between Prokaryotic and Eukaryotic Cells

Prokaryotes and Eukaryotes

Sizes and Metabolism

Cells of the domains of Bacteria and Archaea are **prokaryotes**. Bacteria cells and Archaea cells are much smaller than cells of eukaryotes. Prokaryote cells are usually only 1 to 2 micrometers in diameter, but eukaryotic cells are usually at least 10 times and possibly 100 times larger than prokaryotic cells. Eukaryotic cells are usually 10 to 100 micrometers in diameter. Most prokaryotes are unicellular organisms, although some prokaryotes live in colonies. Because of their large surface-area-to-volume ratios, prokaryotes have a very high metabolic rate. **Eukaryotic cells** are much larger than prokaryotic cells. Due to their larger sizes, they have a much smaller surface-area-to-volume ratio and consequently have much lower metabolic rates.

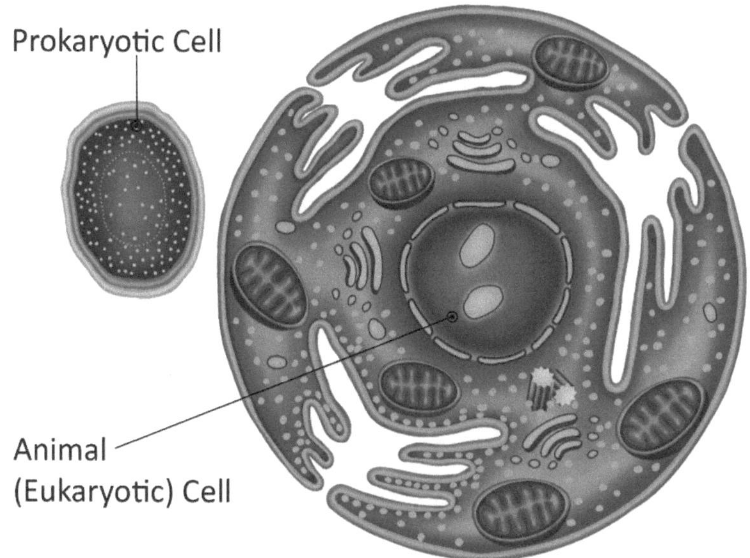

Review Video: Eukaryotic and Prokaryotic Cells
Visit mometrix.com/academy and enter code: 231438

Review Video: Cell Structure
Visit mometrix.com/academy and enter code: 591293

Membrane-Bound Organelles

Prokaryotic cells are much simpler than eukaryotic cells. Prokaryote cells do not have a nucleus due to their small size and their DNA is located in the center of the cell in a region referred to as a **nucleoid**. Eukaryote cells have a **nucleus** bound by a double membrane. Eukaryotic cells typically have hundreds or thousands of additional **membrane-bound organelles** that are independent of the cell membrane. Prokaryotic cells do not have any membrane-bound organelles that are independent of the cell membrane. Once again, this is probably due to the much larger size of the eukaryotic cells. The organelles of eukaryotes give them much higher levels of intracellular division than is possible in prokaryotic cells.

Cell Walls

Not all cells have cell walls, but most prokaryotes have cell walls. The cell walls of organisms from the domain Bacteria differ from the cell walls of the organisms from the domain Archaea. Some eukaryotes, such as some fungi, some algae, and plants, have cell walls that differ from the cell walls of the Bacteria and Archaea domains. The main difference between the cell walls of different domains or kingdoms is the composition of the cell walls. For example, most bacteria have cell walls outside of the plasma membrane that contains the molecule peptidoglycan. **Peptidoglycan** is a large polymer of amino acids and sugars. The peptidoglycan helps maintain the strength of the cell wall. Some of the Archaea cells have cell walls containing the molecule pseudopeptidoglycan, which differs in chemical structure from the peptidoglycan but basically provides the same strength to the cell wall. Some fungi cell walls contain **chitin**. The cell walls of diatoms, a type of yellow algae, contain silica. Plant cell walls contain cellulose, and woody plants are further strengthened by lignin. Some algae also contain lignin. Animal cells do not have cell walls.

Chromosome Structure

Prokaryote cells have DNA arranged in a **circular structure** that should not be referred to as a chromosome. Due to the small size of a prokaryote cell, the DNA material is simply located near the center of the cell in a region called the nucleoid. A prokaryotic cell may also contain tiny rings of DNA called plasmids. Prokaryote cells lack histone proteins, and therefore the DNA is not actually packaged into chromosomes. Prokaryotes reproduce by binary fission, while eukaryotes reproduce by mitosis with the help of **linear chromosomes** and histone proteins. During mitosis, the chromatin is tightly wound on the histone proteins and packaged as a chromosome. The DNA in a eukaryotic cell is located in the membrane-bound nucleus.

Review Video: Chromosomes
Visit mometrix.com/academy and enter code: 132083

Structure and Function of Cells and Organelles

Cells and Organelles of Plant Cells and Animal Cells

Plant cells and animal cells both have a nucleus, cytoplasm, cell membrane, ribosomes, mitochondria, endoplasmic reticulum, Golgi apparatus, and vacuoles. Plant cells have only one or two extremely large vacuoles. Animal cells typically have several small vacuoles. Plant cells have chloroplasts for photosynthesis and use this process to produce their own food, distinguishing plants as **autotrophs**. Animal cells do not have chloroplasts and therefore cannot use photosynthesis to produce their own food. Instead animal cells rely on other sources for food, which classifies them as **heterotrophs**. Animal cells have centrioles, which are used to help organize microtubules and in in cell division, but only some plant cells have centrioles. Additionally, plant cells have a rectangular and more rigid shape due to the cell wall, while animal cells have more of a circular shape because they lack a cell wall.

Review Video: Difference Between Plant and Animal Cells
Visit mometrix.com/academy and enter code: 115568

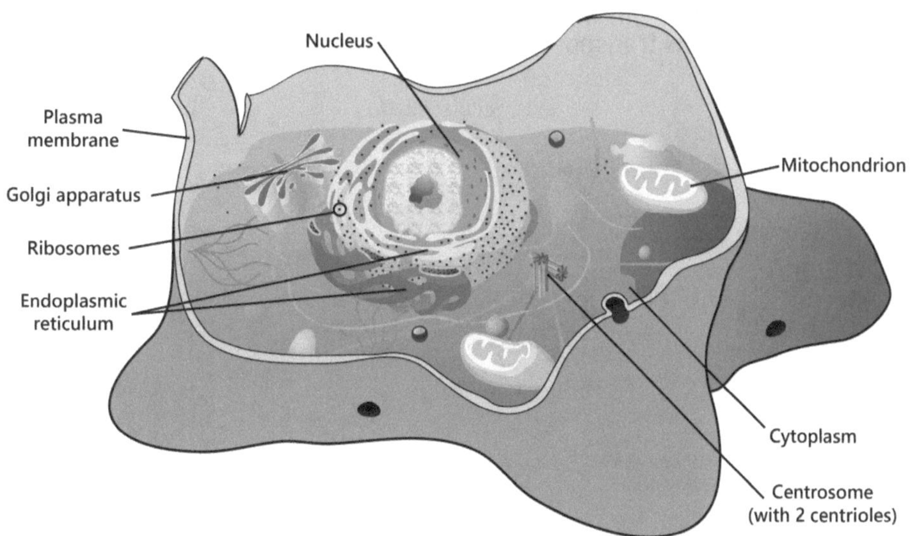

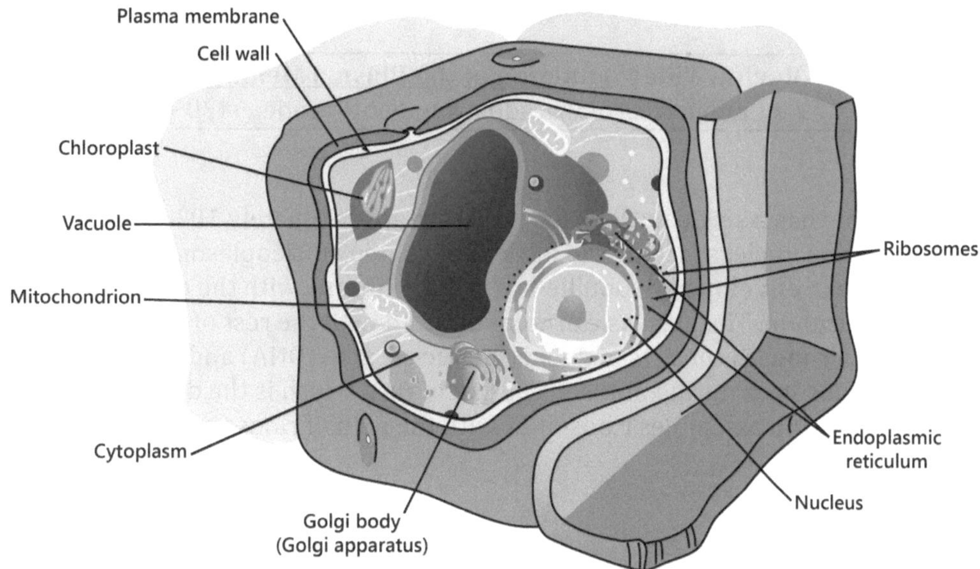

Cell Membranes

The **cell membrane**, also referred to as the plasma membrane, is a thin semipermeable membrane of lipids and proteins. The cell membrane isolates the cell from its external environment while still enabling the cell to communicate with that outside environment. It consists of a phospholipid bilayer, or double layer, with the hydrophilic ("water-loving") ends of the outer layer facing the external environment, the inner layer facing the inside of the cell, and the hydrophobic ("water-fearing") ends facing each other. Cholesterol in the cell membrane adds stiffness and flexibility. Glycolipids help the cell to recognize other cells of the organisms. The proteins in the cell membrane help give the cells shape. Special proteins help the cell communicate with its external environment, while other proteins transport molecules across the cell membrane.

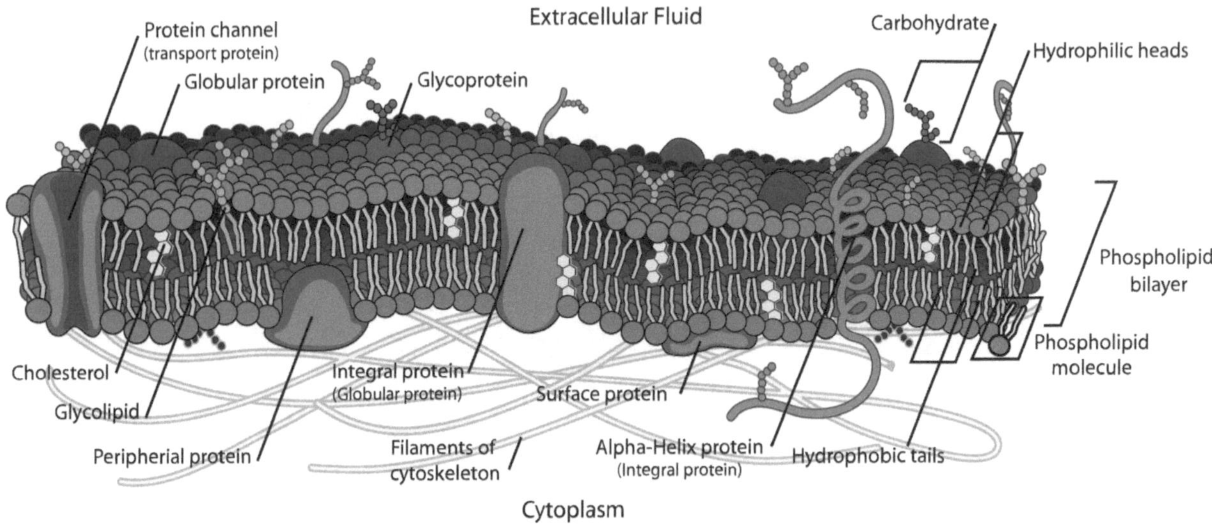

Review Video: Function of the Plasma Membrane
Visit mometrix.com/academy and enter code: 943095

NUCLEUS

Typically, a eukaryote has a single nucleus that takes up approximately 10% of the volume of the cell. Components of the nucleus include the nuclear envelope, nucleoplasm, chromatin, and nucleolus. The **nuclear envelope** is a double-layered membrane with the outer layer connected to the endoplasmic reticulum. The nucleus can communicate with the rest of the cell through several nuclear pores. The chromatin consists of deoxyribonucleic acid (DNA) and histones that are packaged into chromosomes during mitosis. The **nucleolus**, which is the dense central portion of the nucleus, produced and assembles ribosomes with the help of ribosomal RNA and proteins.

Functions of the nucleus include the storage of genetic material, production of ribosomes, and transcription of ribonucleic acid (RNA).

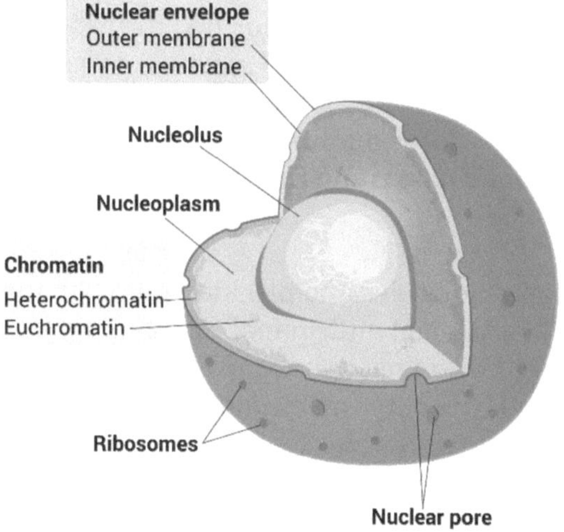

Review Video: Nucleic Acids
Visit mometrix.com/academy and enter code: 503931

Chloroplasts

Chloroplasts are large organelles that are enclosed in a double membrane. Discs called **thylakoids** are arranged in stacks called **grana** (singular, *granum*). The thylakoids have chlorophyll molecules on their surfaces. **Stromal lamellae** separate the thylakoid stacks. Sugars are formed in the stroma, which is the inner portion of the chloroplast. Chloroplasts perform photosynthesis and make food in the form of sugars for the plant. The light reaction stage of photosynthesis occurs in the grana, and the dark reaction stage of photosynthesis occurs in the stroma. Chloroplasts have their own DNA and can reproduce by fission independently.

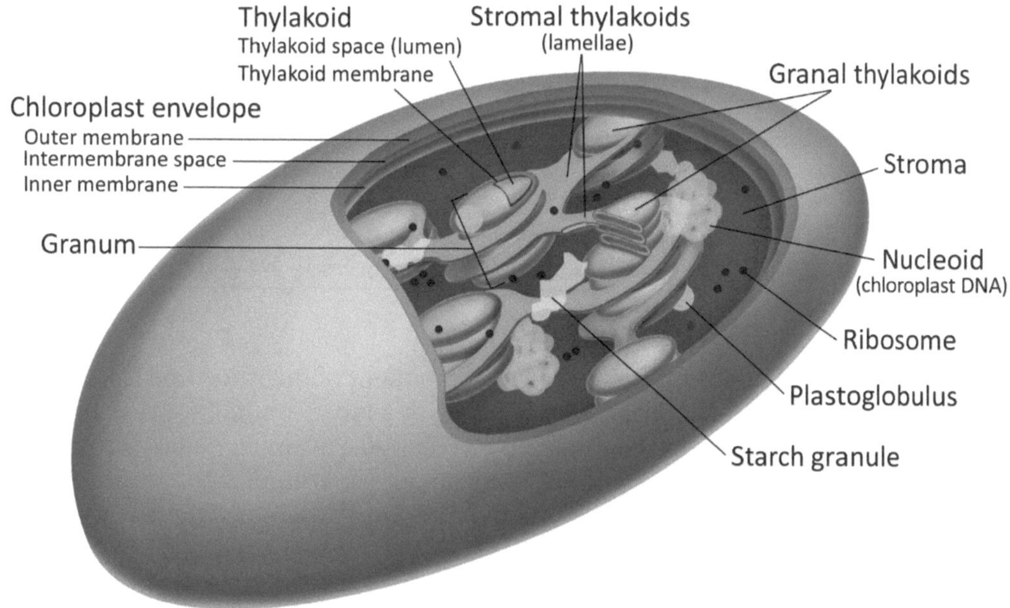

Plastids

Plastids are major organelles found in plants and algae that are used to synthesize and store food. Because plastids can differentiate, there are many forms of plastids. Specialized plastids can store pigments, starches, fats, or proteins. Two examples of plastids are amyloplasts and chloroplasts. **Amyloplasts** are the plastids that store the starch formed from long chains of glucose produced during photosynthesis. Amyloplasts synthesize and store the starch granules through the polymerization of glucose. When needed, amyloplasts also convert these starch granules back into sugar. Fruits and potato tubers have large numbers of amyloplasts. **Chloroplasts** can synthesize and store starch. Interestingly, amyloplasts can redifferentiate and transform into chloroplasts.

Mitochondria

Mitochondria break down sugar molecules and produce energy in the form of molecules of adenosine triphosphate (ATP). Both plant and animal cells contain mitochondria. Mitochondria are enclosed in a bilayer semi-membrane of phospholipids and proteins. The intermembrane space is the space between the two layers. The outer membrane has proteins called porins, which allow small molecules through. The inner membrane contains proteins that aid in the synthesis of ATP. The matrix consists of enzymes that help synthesize ATP. Mitochondria have their own DNA and can reproduce by fission independently. Mitochondria also help to maintain calcium concentrations, form blood components and hormones, and are involved in activating cell death pathways.

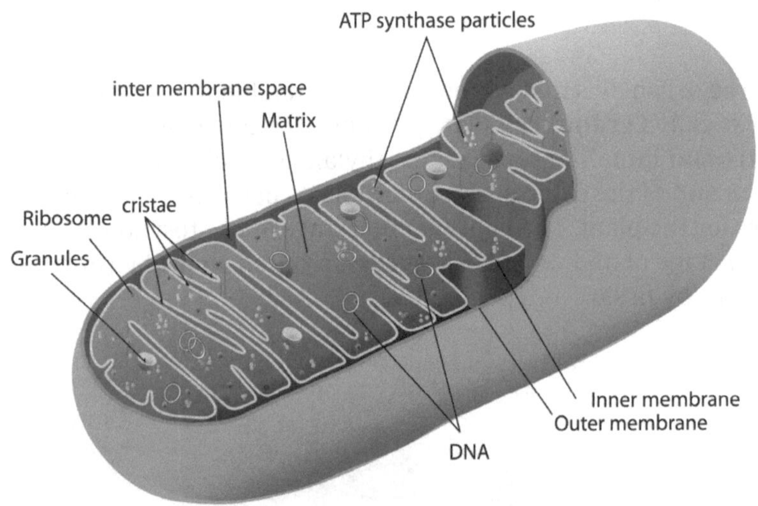

Review Video: Mitochondria
Visit mometrix.com/academy and enter code: 444287

Ribosomes

A **ribosome** consists of RNA and proteins. The RNA component of the ribosome is known as ribosomal RNA (rRNA). Ribosomes consist of two subunits, a large subunit and a small subunit. Few ribosomes are free in the cell. Most of the ribosomes in the cell are embedded in the rough endoplasmic reticulum located near the nucleus. Ribosomes are protein factories and translate the code of DNA into proteins by assembling long chains of amino acids. **Messenger RNA** (mRNA) is used by the ribosome to generate a specific protein sequence, while **transfer RNA** (tRNA) collects the needed amino acids and delivers them to the ribosome.

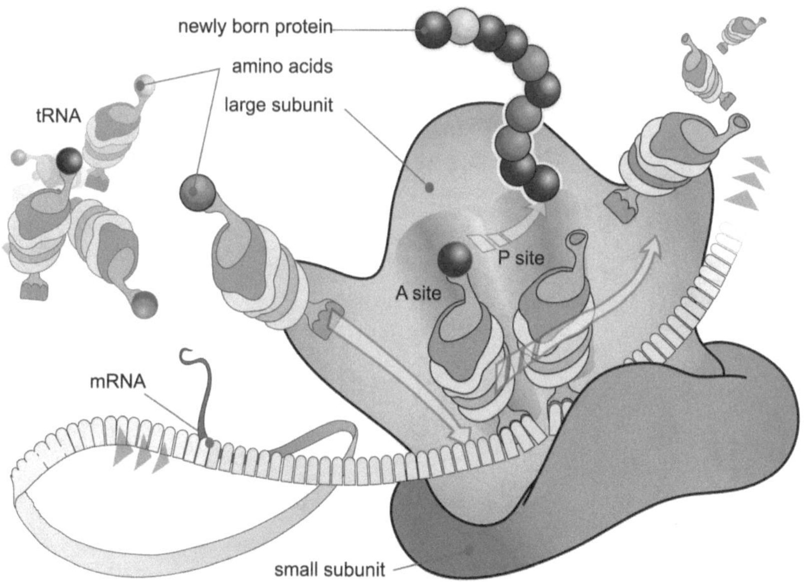

Golgi Apparatus

The **Golgi apparatus**, also called the Golgi body or Golgi complex, is a stack of flattened membranes called **cisternae** that package, ship, and distribute macromolecules such as carbohydrates, proteins, and lipids in shipping containers called **vesicles**. It also helps modify proteins and lipids before they are shipped. Most Golgi apparatuses have six to eight cisternae. Each Golgi apparatus has four regions: the cis region, the endo region, the medial region, and the trans region. Transfer vesicles from the rough endoplasmic reticulum (ER) enter at the cis region, and secretory vesicles leave the Golgi apparatus from the trans region.

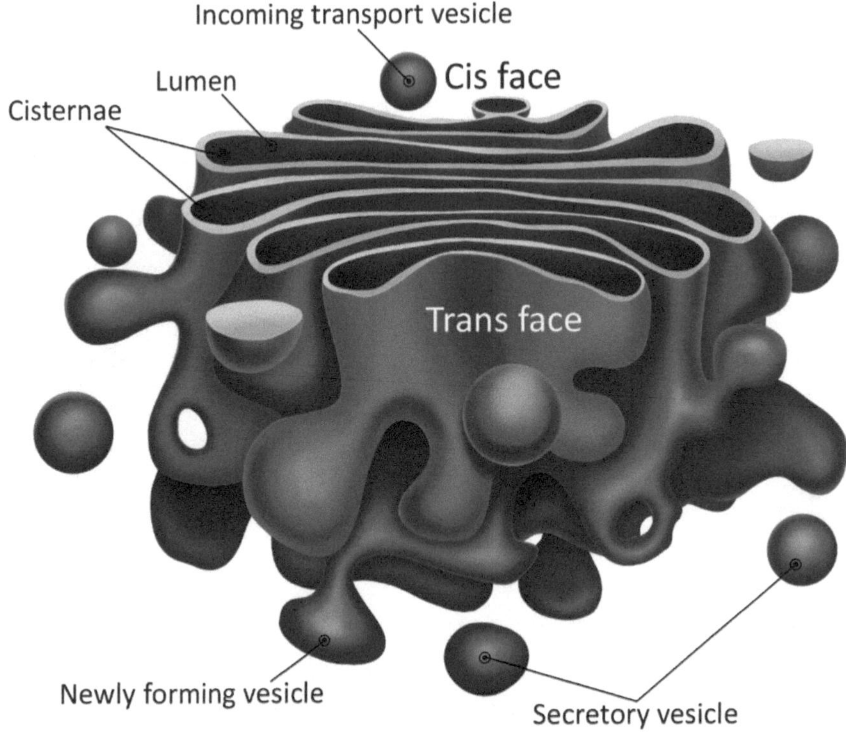

Cytoskeleton

The **cytoskeleton** is a scaffolding system located in the cytoplasm. The cytoskeleton consists of elongated organelles made of proteins called microtubules, microfilaments, and intermediate filaments. These organelles provide shape, support, and the ability to move. These structures also assist in moving the chromosomes during mitosis. Microtubules and microfilaments help transport materials throughout the cell and are the major components in cilia and flagella.

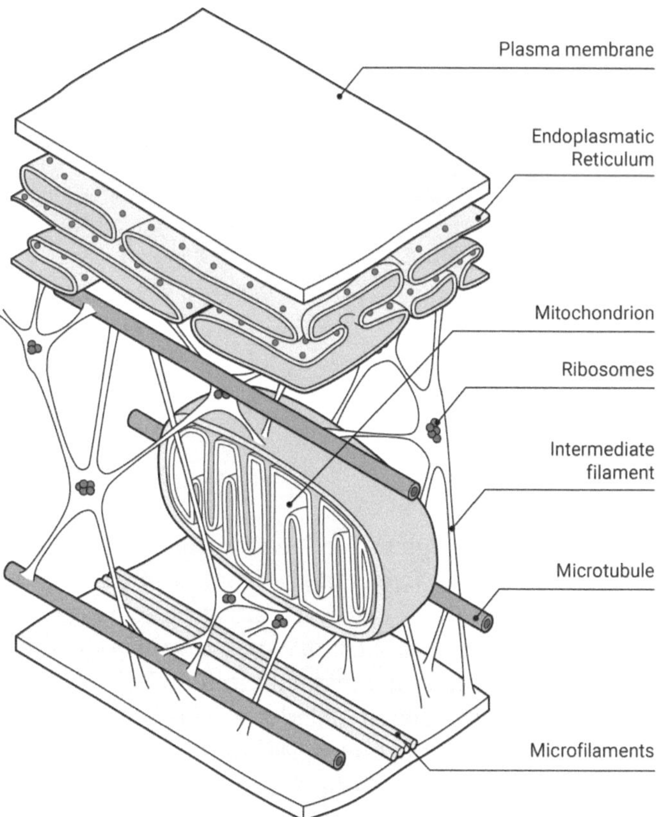

Cellular Homeostasis

Selective Permeability

The cell membrane, or plasma membrane, has selective permeability with regard to size, charge, and solubility. With regard to molecule size, the cell membrane allows only small molecules to diffuse through it. Oxygen and water molecules are small and typically can pass through the cell membrane. The charge of the ions on the cell's surface also either attracts or repels ions. Ions with like charges are repelled, and ions with opposite charges are attracted to the cell's surface. Molecules that are soluble in phospholipids can usually pass through the cell membrane. Many molecules are not able to diffuse the cell membrane, and, if needed, those molecules must be moved through by active transport and vesicles.

Active and Passive Transport

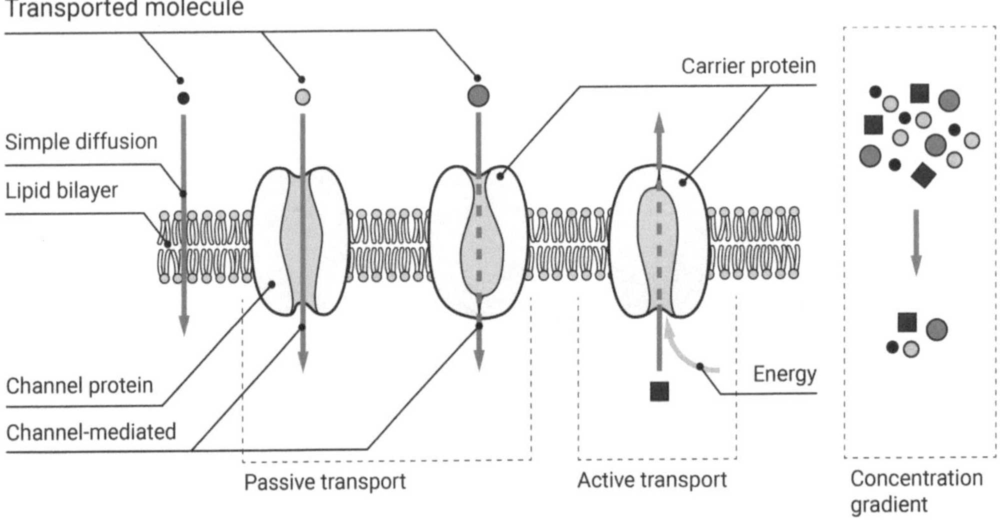

Cells can move materials in and out through the cell membrane by active and passive transport. In **passive transport**, the molecules diffuse across the cell membrane by osmosis. These molecules are moving from a region where they have a high concentration to a region where the concentration is lower. In passive transport, the molecules move across the cell membrane without the cell expending any extra energy. Diffusion and facilitated diffusion are considered passive transport. **Facilitated diffusion** occurs when molecules are helped across the membrane by certain proteins called channel proteins or carrier proteins. Because facilitated diffusion is still from a region of high to low concentration, it does not require additional energy and is therefore a type of passive transport. In active transport, molecules are forcibly moved from regions where the concentration is low into a region where the concentration is higher. Carrier proteins must carry these ions and molecules, and this requires an expenditure of energy. Some ions are actively pumped across the cell membrane by proteins. Sodium ions are pumped out of cell, and potassium ions are pumped into the cell in this manner.

> **Review Video: Passive Transport: Diffusion and Osmosis**
> Visit mometrix.com/academy and enter code: 642038

Water Movement to Maintain Internal Environments of Cells

Cells must maintain their water balance for **homeostasis**. If cells have too little water, wastes and poisons can build up in the cells. If cells have too much water, the chemicals in the cells may be diluted. Water is moved in and out of cells by **osmosis**. Because osmosis is a type of passive transport, the cell cannot actually control this diffusion of water in and out of the cells. The amount of water that diffuses into or out of cells depends on the cell's environment. When the cell's concentration of water and dissolved solids equals that of its environment, the cells are **isotonic** with their environment. Cells with a lower concentration of water than their environment tend to rapidly gain water by osmosis. These cells are **hypotonic** with their environment. Cells with a higher concentration of water than their environment tend to rapidly lose water by osmosis. The cells are **hypertonic** with their environment. If cells are hypotonic or hypertonic, they must expend energy to maintain the proper water balance.

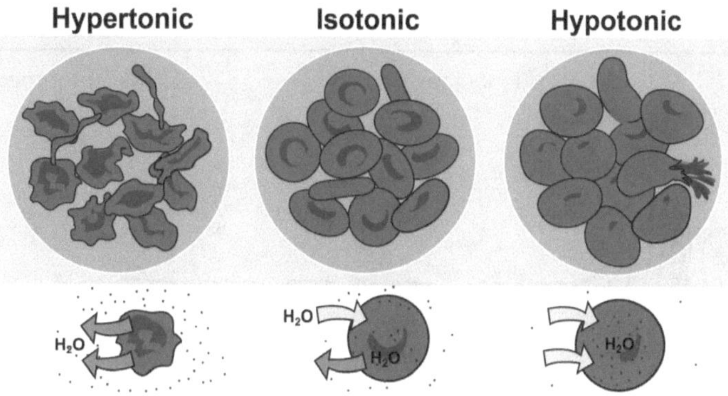

Use of Cell Surface Proteins and Cell Communication

In order to maintain a stable internal environment, cells need to send and receive signals from the external environment. Cells have specialized surface proteins called **receptors** embedded in the cell membrane that allow them to communicate with this external environment. Some surface proteins are exposed to the external side of the membrane. Some surface proteins allow entry to specific materials, and others trigger chemical signals inside the cell. Because these proteins have attached carbohydrates, they are called **glycoproteins**. Due to the cholesterol in the cell membrane, fat-soluble materials can pass straight through the membrane, but water-soluble materials cannot diffuse. Sodium, calcium, and potassium must use these specialized surface proteins to gain entry to the cell. These surface proteins bind to specific chemicals in the materials seeking access to the cell. This triggers a chemical signal to the interior of the cell.

Exocytosis and Endocytosis

Larger particles or groups of particles can be transported whole across the cell membrane by being packaged in a piece of cell membrane. **Endocytosis** is the process by which large particles are moved into the cell, and **exocytosis** is the process by which large molecules are moved out of the cell. The three main types of endocytosis are phagocytosis, pinocytosis, and receptor-mediated endocytosis. **Phagocytosis**, or "cell eating," is the process by which large solid particles are engulfed. **Pinocytosis**, or "cell drinking," is the process by which liquids and dissolved substances are surrounded by small sacs of cell membrane. **Receptor-mediated endocytosis** is the process by which molecules enter cells through receptor molecules on the cell membrane.

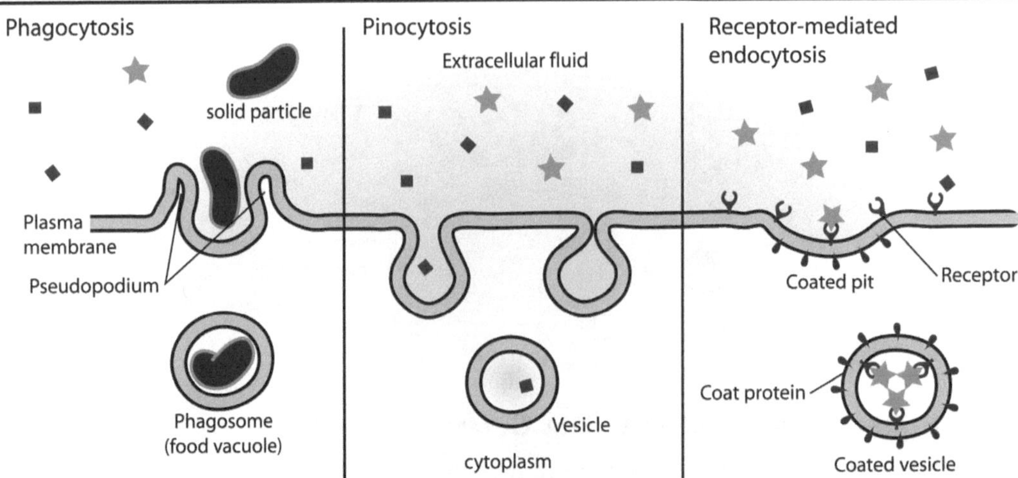

Hormone Action and Feedback

In order to maintain homeostasis, the endocrine system often employs negative-feedback inhibition or positive-feedback regulation. In **negative-feedback inhibition**, an increase in an output of a reaction to a stimulus triggers a decrease in the stimulus, which in turn causes a decrease in the original output. In **positive-feedback regulation**, an increase in an output leads to further increase of the stimulus. An example of negative-feedback inhibition is the release of the hormones insulin and glucagon to maintain the level of glucose in the blood.

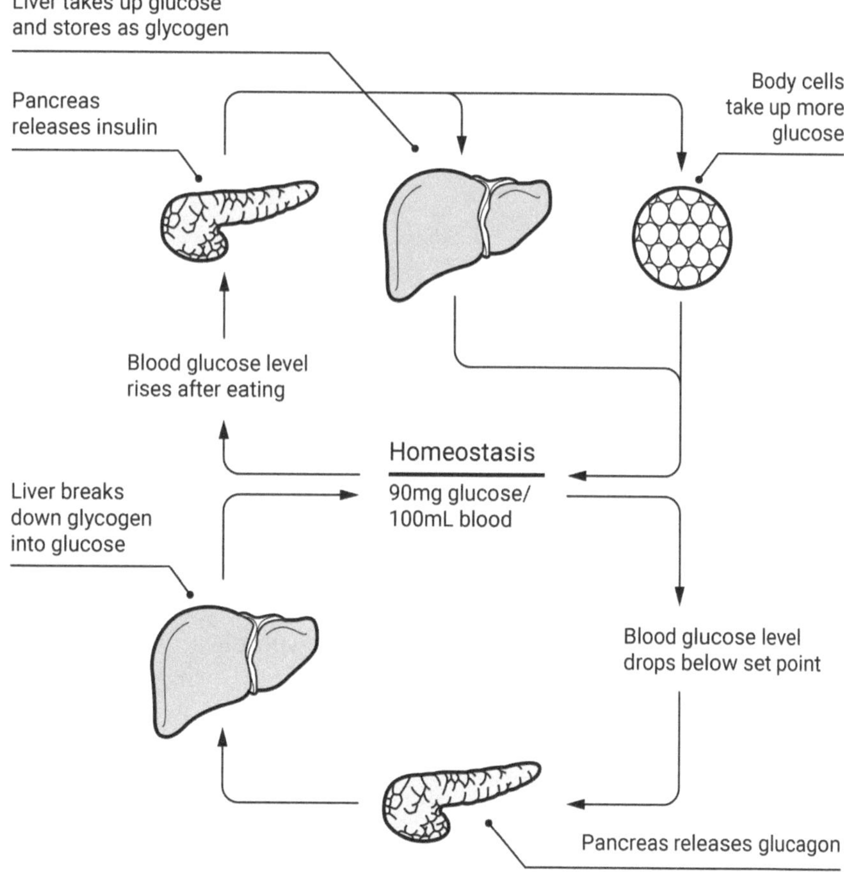

Cell Cycle and Cellular Division

Cell Cycle Stages

The cell cycle consists of three stages: interphase, mitosis, and cytokinesis. **Interphase** is the longest stage of the cell cycle and involves the cell growing and making a copy of its DNA. Cells typically spend more than 90% of the cell cycle in interphase. Interphase includes two growth phases called G_1 and G_2. The order of interphase is the first growth cycle, **GAP 1** (G_1 phase), followed by the **synthesis phase** (S), and ending with the second growth phase, **GAP 2** (G_2 phase). During the G_1 phase of interphase, the cell increases the number of organelles by forming diploid cells. During the S phase of interphase, the DNA is replicated, and the chromosomes are doubled.

During the G_2 phase of interphase, the cell synthesizes needed proteins and organelles, continues to increase in size, and prepares for mitosis. Once the G_2 phase ends, mitosis can begin.

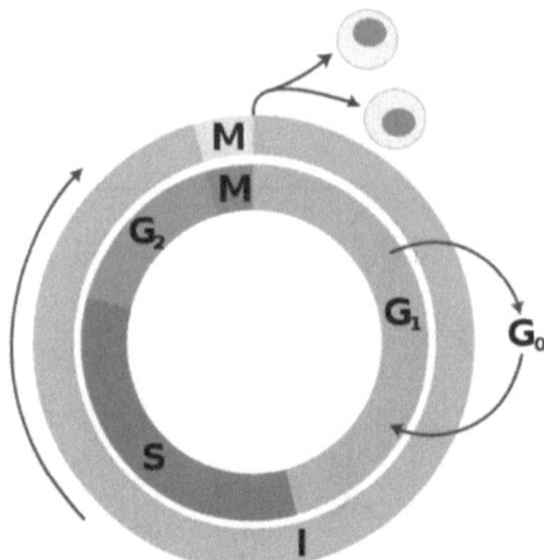

Mitosis

Mitosis is the asexual process of cell division. During mitosis, one parent cell divides into two identical daughter cells. Mitosis is used for growth, repair, and replacement of cells. Some unicellular organisms reproduce asexually by mitosis. Some multicellular organisms can reproduce by fragmentation or budding, which involves mitosis. Mitosis consists of four phases: prophase, metaphase, anaphase, and telophase. During **prophase**, the spindle fibers appear and the DNA is condensed and packaged as chromosomes that become visible. The nuclear membrane also breaks down, and the nucleolus disappears. During **metaphase**, the spindle apparatus is formed and the centromeres of the chromosomes line up on the equatorial plane. During **anaphase**, the centromeres divide and the two chromatids separate and are pulled toward the opposite poles of the cell. During **telophase**, the spindle fibers disappear, the nuclear membrane reforms, and the DNA in the chromatids is decondensed.

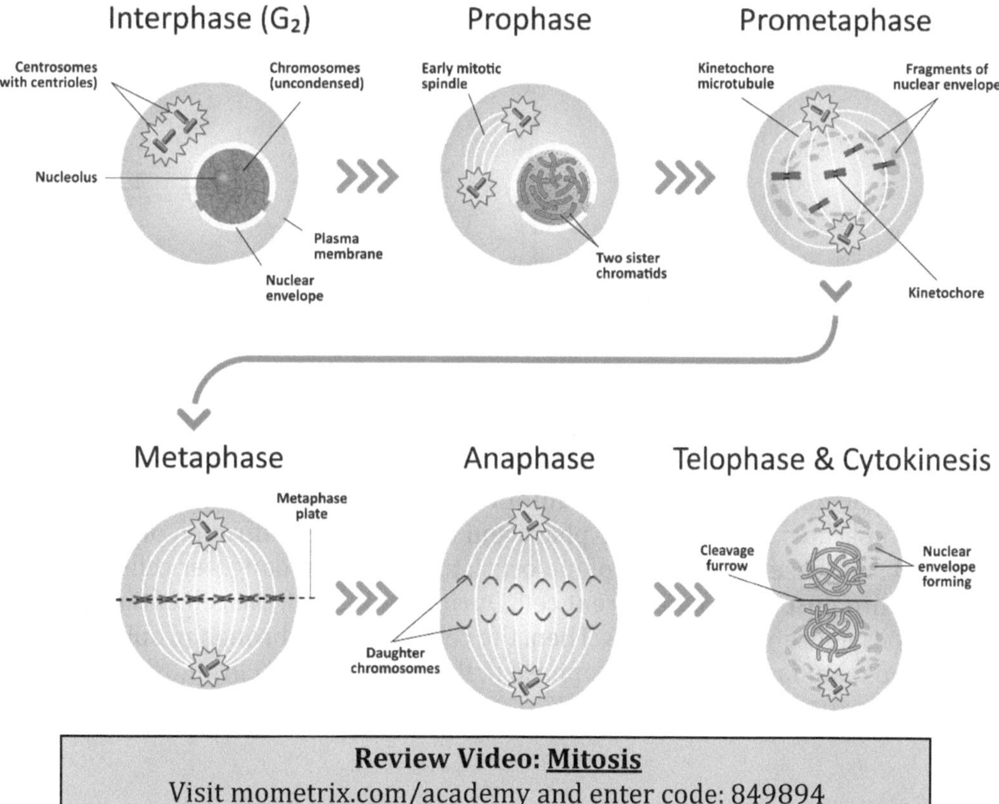

Review Video: Mitosis
Visit mometrix.com/academy and enter code: 849894

Cytokinesis

Cytokinesis is the dividing of the cytoplasm and cell membrane by the pinching of a cell into two new daughter cells at the end of mitosis. This occurs at the end of telophase when the actin filaments in the cytoskeleton form a contractile ring that narrows and divides the cell. In plant cells, a cell plate forms across the phragmoplast, which is the center of the spindle apparatus. In animal cells, as the contractile ring narrows, the cleavage furrow forms. Eventually, the contractile ring narrows down to the spindle apparatus joining the two cells and the cells eventually divide. Diagrams of the cleavage furrow of an animal cell and cell plate of a plant are shown below.

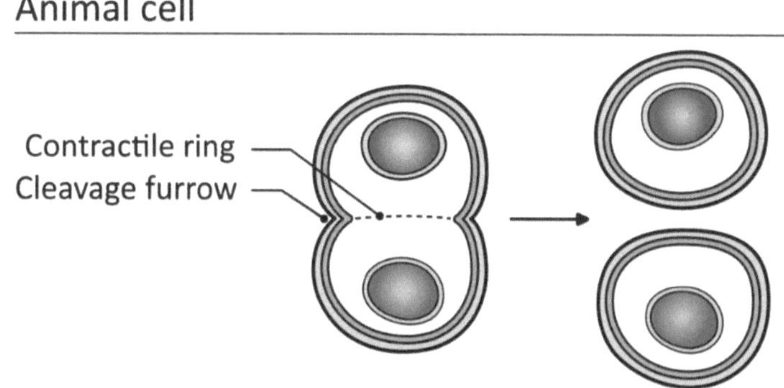

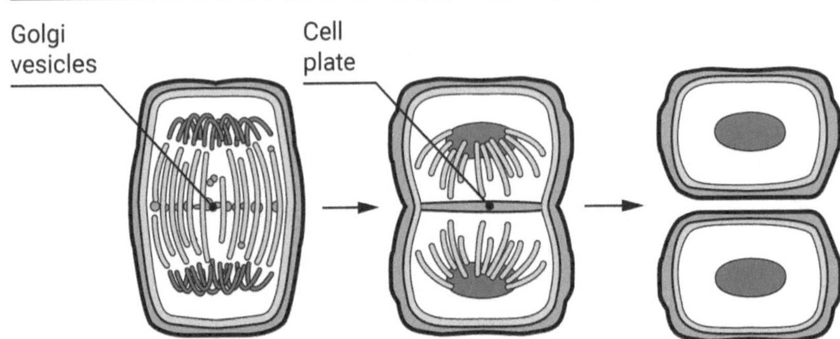

Meiosis

Meiosis is a type of cell division in which the number of chromosomes is reduced by half. Meiosis produces gametes, or egg and sperm cells. Meiosis occurs in two successive stages, which consist of a first mitotic division followed by a second mitotic division. During **meiosis I**, or the first meiotic division, the cell replicates its DNA in interphase and then continues through prophase I, metaphase I, anaphase I, and telophase I. At the end of meiosis I, there are two daughter cells that have the same number of chromosomes as the parent cell. During **meiosis II**, the cell enters a brief interphase but does not replicate its DNA. Then, the cell continues through prophase II, metaphase II, anaphase II, and telophase II. During prophase II, the unduplicated chromosomes split. At the end of telophase II, there are four daughter cells that have half the number of chromosomes as the parent cell.

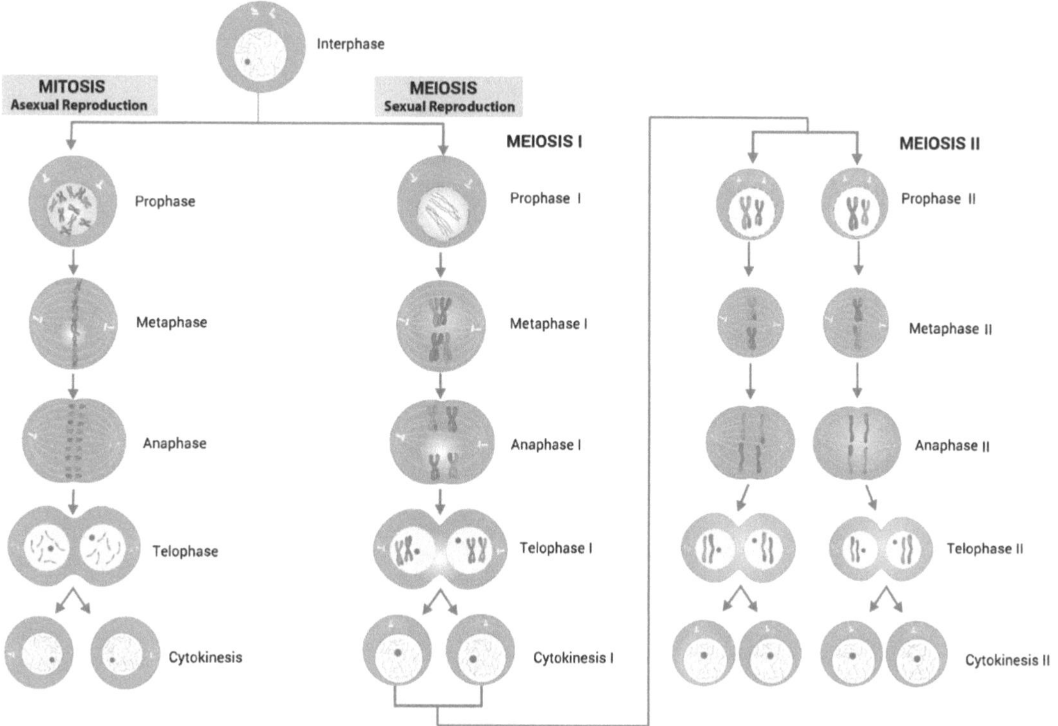

Review Video: Meiosis
Visit mometrix.com/academy and enter code: 247334

Cell Cycle Checkpoints

During the cell cycle, the cell goes through three checkpoints to ensure that the cell is dividing properly at each phase, that it is the appropriate time for division, and that the cell has not been damaged. The **first checkpoint** is at the end of the G_1 phase just before the cell undergoes the S phase, or synthesis. At this checkpoint, a cell may continue with cell division, delay the division, or rest. This **resting phase** is called G_0. In animal cells, the G_1 checkpoint is called **restriction.** Proteins called cyclin D and cyclin E, which are dependent on enzymes cyclin-dependent kinase 4 and cyclin-dependent kinase 2 (CDK4 and CDK2), respectively, largely control this first checkpoint. The **second checkpoint** is at the end of the G_2 phase just before the cell begins prophase during mitosis. The protein cyclin A, which is dependent on the enzyme CDK2, largely controls this checkpoint. During mitosis, the **third checkpoint** occurs at metaphase to check that the

Science

chromosomes are lined up along the equatorial plane. This checkpoint is largely controlled by cyclin B, which is dependent upon the enzyme CDK1.

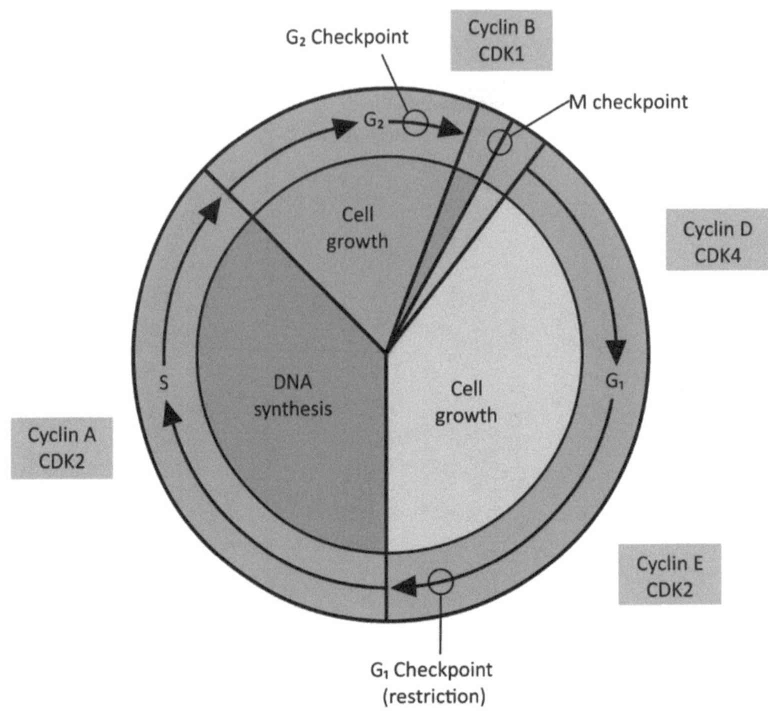

Nucleic Acids

Nucleotide Structure

A **nucleotide**, whether DNA or RNA, contains three components: a phosphate group, a ringed, five-carbon sugar (deoxyribose in DNA, ribose in RNA), and a nitrogen-containing base. The **phosphate group** binds to one side of the **ringed, five-carbon sugar**. The **nitrogen-containing base** binds to the opposite side of the ringed, five-carbon sugar. A nucleotide strand is formed by covalently linking the phosphate groups of the nucleotides into a linear sequence.

Nitrogenous base
(Adenine)

Phosphate
group

Five-carbon sugar
(Deoxyribose)

DNA AND RNA

STRUCTURAL SIMILARITIES

Structural similarities between DNA and RNA:

- DNA and RNA are both **nucleic acids** composed of nucleotides made up of a sugar, a base, and a phosphate molecule.
- DNA and RNA have three of their four bases in common: guanine, cytosine, and adenine.

Review Video: DNA Vs. RNA
Visit mometrix.com/academy and enter code: 184871

STRUCTURAL, LOCATIONAL, AND FUNCTIONAL DIFFERENCES

Structural differences between DNA and RNA:

- DNA contains the base thymine, but RNA replaces thymine with uracil.
- DNA contains the sugar deoxyribose, but RNA contains the sugar ribose.
- DNA is double stranded, but RNA is single stranded.

Locational – DNA is located in the nucleus and mitochondria. RNA is found in the nucleus, ribosomes, and cytoplasm.

Functional – DNA contains the genetic blueprint and instructions for the cell. RNA carries out those instructions and synthesizes proteins.

TYPES AND FUNCTIONS OF RNA

Types of RNA include ribosomal RNA (rRNA), transfer RNA (tRNA), and messenger RNA (mRNA).

- **rRNA**: forms the RNA component of the ribosome. It is evolutionarily conserved, which means it can be used to study relationships in organisms.
- **mRNA**: used by the ribosome to generate proteins (translation). The mRNA contains three-nucleotide "codons" that code for specific amino acids in a protein sequence.
- **tRNA**: functions in translation by transferring an amino acid to the corresponding codon on the mRNA strand.

Review Video: DNA
Visit mometrix.com/academy and enter code: 639552

COMPLEMENTARY BASE PAIRING

According to **Chargaff's rule**, a DNA molecule always has a 1:1 ratio of purine to pyrimidine within it. The amount of adenine always equals the amount of thymine, and the amount of guanine always equals the amount of cytosine. (Note that the same rule holds for RNA, but the thymine is replaced with uracil.) In DNA, adenine always pairs with thymine, and guanine always pairs with cytosine. In RNA, adenine always pairs with uracil, and guanine always pairs with cytosine. The pairs are bonded together with hydrogen bonds.

DOUBLE HELIX STRUCTURE OF DNA

Double-stranded DNA consists of two complementary strands that adopt the shape of a double helix, which resembles a twisted ladder. The "sides" of the ladder are the sugar-phosphate backbones of the complementary strands. The "rungs" of the ladder are the nitrogenous bases, which are held together (base paired) by hydrogen bonds between the complementary nitrogenous bases in the opposite strand. In DNA, **adenine** (A) base pairs with **thymine** (T) and **guanine** (G) base pairs with **cytosine** (C). DNA also has an antiparallel structure, consisting of a 5' end and a 3' end, where the two strands of the DNA run in opposite directions for one another. The two ends of the DNA strand are coined 5' or 3' based on the specific carbon atom within the purine or pyrimidine ring that makes up the deoxyribose sugar. The 5' end of a DNA strand has a free phosphate group attached to the 5'-carbon atom of the deoxyribose sugar, while the 3' end of DNA has a free hydroxyl group at the 3'-carbon.

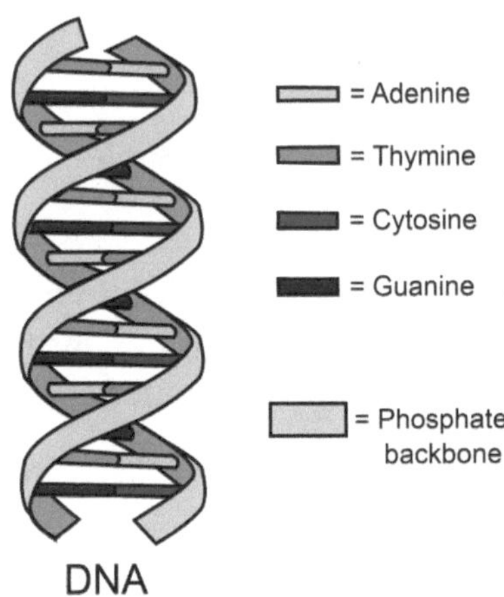

Organization of Prokaryotic DNA

Prokaryotes lack a nucleus and therefore prokaryotic DNA is organized primarily into a central loop contained in the cytoplasm. Prokaryotes may also contain smaller loops of DNA known as **plasmids** that contain other genes. Most prokaryotes lack histones, but Archae are an example of prokaryotes that do contain histones.

Organization of Eukaryotic DNA

Eukaryotes have a nucleus with multiple chromosomes, each containing a tightly-compacted, double-helix DNA molecule. The structural sub-components of chromosomes include histones, nucleosomes, and chromatin.

- **Histones** are positively-charged, DNA-binding proteins.
- A **nucleosome** is composed of eight histone proteins around which approximately 146 base pairs of DNA are wrapped. The nucleosome is often called a "beads on a string" structure.
- **Chromatin** is made up of compacted nucleosomes.
- **Chromosomes** are made up of compacted chromatin.

RNA is also thought to play a role in chromatin structure.

Telomeres

Eukaryotic chromosomes have **telomeres** located at their tips. Telomeres are repetitive sequences of DNA that maintain the ends of the linear chromosomes and keep those ends from deteriorating.

DNA Replication

DNA replication begins when the double strands of the parent DNA molecule are unwound and unzipped. The enzyme **helicase** separates the two strands by breaking the hydrogen bonds between the base pairs that make up the rungs of the twisted ladder. These two single strands of

DNA are called the **replication fork.** Each separate DNA strand provides a template for the complementary DNA bases, G with C and A with T. The opposite ends of DNA are called the 5' and 3' ends. After the DNA is separated, the enzyme **RNA primase** lays down an RNA primer that the enzyme **DNA polymerase** binds to initiate replication. DNA polymerase only synthesizes DNA from the 5' end towards the 3' end. Of the two strands open during replication, the strand with the 3' end will be replicated as a single, continuous strand, also known as the **leading strand**. The strand with the 5' end, which runs away from the fork is known as the **lagging strand**, and will be replicated into shorter, unlinked segments known as Okizaki fragments. After bases are joined to the complementary base, the enzyme **exonuclease** removes the RNA primers used to initiate replication of the two strands. A separate DNA polymerase fills in gaps after the RNA primer is removed. The Okizaki fragments are joined by the enzyme DNA ligase.

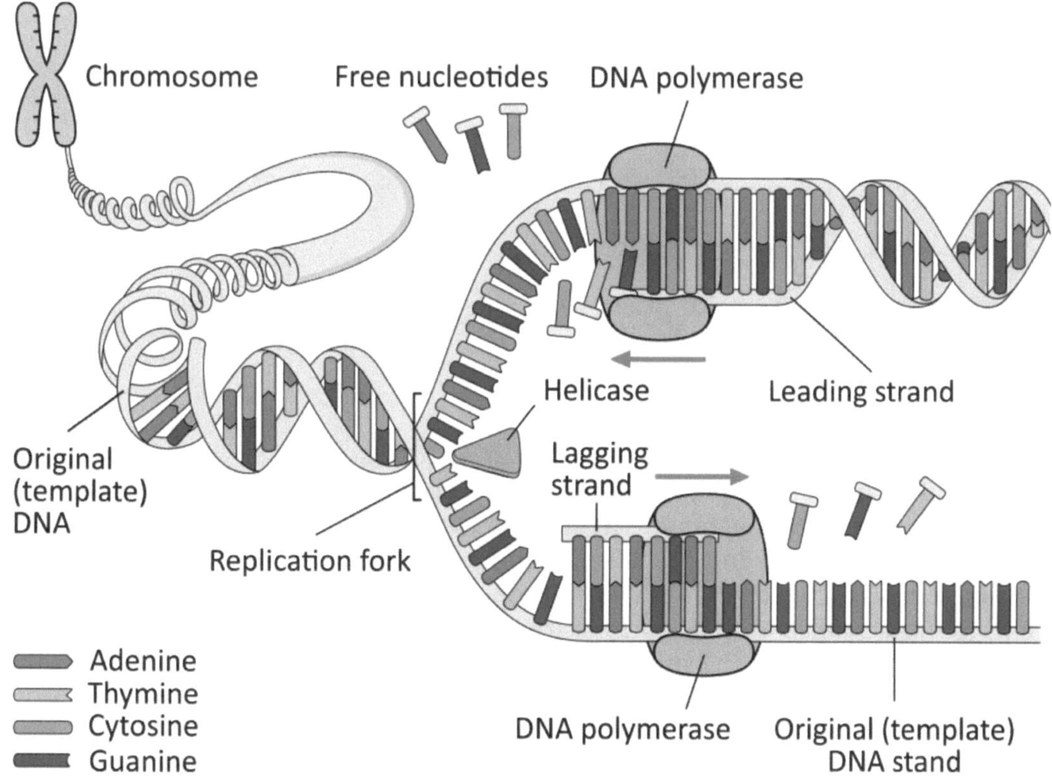

Protein Synthesis

Transcription

Transcription is the process by which a segment of DNA is copied onto a working blueprint called RNA. Each gene has a special region called a **promoter** that guides the beginning of the transcription process. **RNA polymerase** unwinds the DNA at the promoter region and makes an RNA copy of the DNA gene by adding the **complementary nucleotides**, G with C, C with G, T with A, and A with U. This forms a single strand of messenger RNA or mRNA.

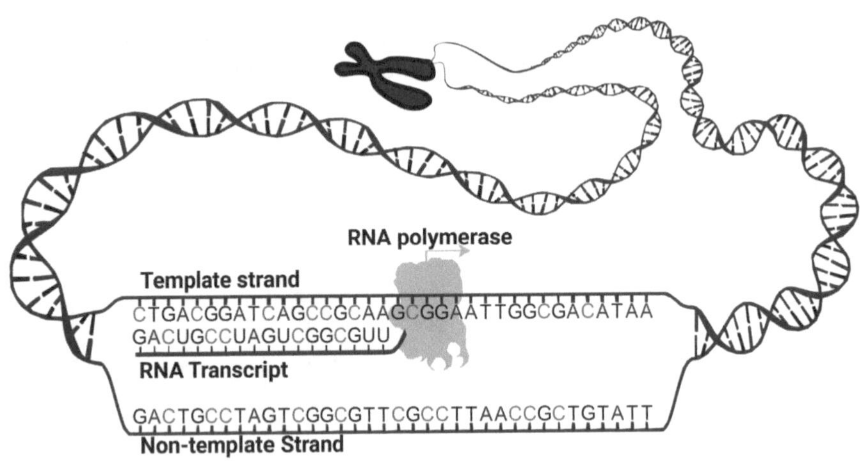

Processing mRNA

In addition to being transcribed, the mRNA must also be processed. First, a 5' cap (modified guanine nucleotide) is added, which helps promote ribosome recognition and preventing mRNA degradation. Second, a string of adenosine ribonucleotides are added to the 3' end of the mRNA, forming a structure known as a **poly(A) tail**. The poly(A) tail helps prevent mRNA degradation. The mRNA transcript may contain regions that do not code for protein, called **introns**. The regions that do code for protein are called **exons**. If introns are present, they will be removed in a process called splicing by a structure known as the **spliceosome**. After addition of the 5' cap, addition of the poly(A) tail, and splicing, the mRNA is ready for translation.

Translation

Ribosomes synthesize proteins from mRNA in a process called **translation**. The ribosome has three tRNA binding sites—A, P, and E. Translation initiates when the "**A site**" becomes occupied by the tRNA molecule corresponding to the mRNA start codon. The ribosome then moves the first tRNA from the "A site" to the "**P site**." The "A site" is then occupied by the tRNA molecule corresponding to the second mRNA codon. The ribosome then transfers the amino acid on the "P site" tRNA to the amino acid on the "A site" tRNA. The first tRNA, which now has no amino acid, is moved from the "P site" the "**E site**." The second tRNA, complexed to a chain of two amino acids, is moved from the "A site" to the "P site." The "A site" is then occupied by the tRNA corresponding to the third mRNA codon. The "P site" amino acid chain is transferred to the amino acid bound to the "A site" tRNA. The first tRNA then exits from the "E site" and the second and third tRNA molecules shift, opening the "A site" for the next tRNA. The growing amino acid chain continues to be transferred from the "P site" to the "A site" until translation is complete.

Review Video: Amino Acids
Visit mometrix.com/academy and enter code: 190385

Anatomy and Physiology

HIERARCHY OF MULTICELLULAR ORGANISMS

ORGANIZATIONAL HIERARCHY WITHIN MULTICELLULAR ORGANISMS

Cells are the smallest living units of organisms. Tissues are groups of cells that work together to perform a specific function. Organs are groups of tissues that work together to perform a specific function. Organ systems are groups of organs that work together to perform a specific function. An organism is an individual that contains several body systems.

CELLS

Cells are the basic structural units of all living things. Cells are composed of various molecules including proteins, carbohydrates, lipids, and nucleic acids. All animal cells are eukaryotic and have a nucleus, cytoplasm, and a cell membrane. Organelles include mitochondria, ribosomes, endoplasmic reticulum, Golgi apparatuses, and vacuoles. Specialized cells are numerous, including but not limited to, muscle cells, nerve cells, epithelial cells, bone cells, blood cells, and cartilage cells. Cells can be grouped together in tissues to perform specific functions.

TISSUES

Tissues are groups of cells that work together to perform a specific function. Tissues can be grouped into four broad categories: muscle tissue, connective tissue, nerve tissue, and epithelial tissue. Muscle tissue is involved in body movement. **Muscle tissues** can be composed of skeletal muscle cells, cardiac muscle cells, or smooth muscle cells. Skeletal muscles include the muscles commonly called biceps, triceps, hamstrings, and quadriceps. Cardiac muscle tissue is found only in the heart. Smooth muscle tissue provides tension in the blood vessels, controls pupil dilation, and aids in peristalsis. **Connective tissues** include bone tissue, cartilage, tendons, ligaments, fat, blood, and lymph. **Nerve tissue** is located in the brain, spinal cord, and nerves. **Epithelial tissue** makes up the layers of the skin and various membranes. Tissues are grouped together as organs to perform specific functions.

ORGANS AND ORGAN SYSTEMS

Organs are groups of tissues that work together to perform specific functions. **Organ systems** are groups of organs that work together to perform specific functions. Complex animals have several organs that are grouped together in multiple systems. In mammals, there are 11 major organ systems: integumentary system, respiratory system, cardiovascular system, endocrine system, nervous system, immune system, digestive system, excretory system, muscular system, skeletal system, and reproductive system.

Human Anatomy and Physiology

The Three Primary Body Planes

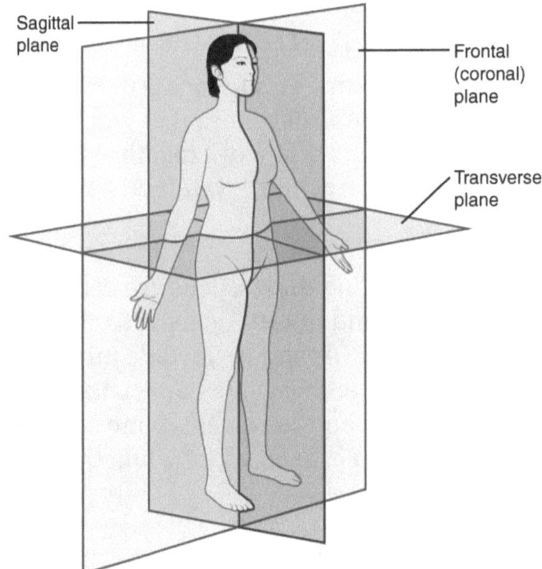

The **transverse (or horizontal) plane** divides the patient's body into upper (*superior*) and lower (*inferior or caudal*) halves.

The **sagittal plane** divides the body, or any body part, vertically into right and left sections. The sagittal plane runs parallel to the midline of the body.

The **coronal (or frontal) plane** divides the body, or any body structure, vertically into front and back (*anterior* and *posterior*) sections. The coronal plane runs vertically through the body and is perpendicular to the sagittal plane.

Cardiovascular System

The main functions of the **cardiovascular system** are gas exchange, the delivery of nutrients and hormones, and waste removal. The cardiovascular system consists primarily of the heart, blood, and blood vessels. The **heart** is a pump that pushes blood through the arteries. **Arteries** are blood vessels that carry blood away from the heart, and **veins** are blood vessels that carry blood back to the heart. The exchange of materials between blood and cells occur in the **capillaries**, which are the smallest of the blood vessels. All vertebrates and a few invertebrates including annelids, squids, and octopuses have a **closed circulatory system**, in which blood is contained in vessels and does not freely fill body cavities. Mammals, birds and crocodilians have a four-chambered heart. Most amphibians and reptiles have a three-chambered heart. Fish have only a two-chambered heart. Arthropods and most mollusks have open circulatory systems, where blood is pumped into an open cavity. Many invertebrates do not have a cardiovascular system. For example, echinoderms have a water vascular system.

Review Video: Functions of the Circulatory System
Visit mometrix.com/academy and enter code: 376581

Review Video: Mnemonics for Heart Anatomy and Physiology
Visit mometrix.com/academy and enter code: 849489

Review Video: Electrical Conduction System of the Heart
Visit mometrix.com/academy and enter code: 624557

Review Video: How the Heart Functions
Visit mometrix.com/academy and enter code: 569724

Heart Chambers and Valves

There are four chambers of the heart that have valves separating them and regulating a one-way flow of blood between the chambers.

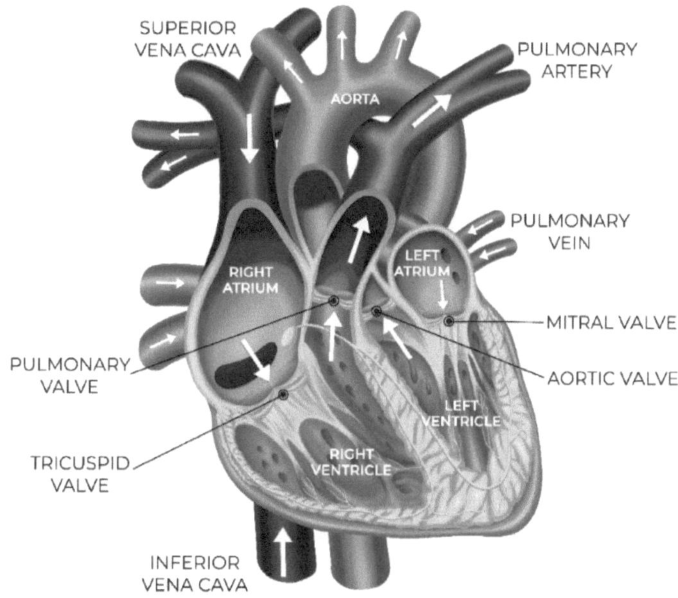

Respiratory System

The function of the **respiratory system** is to move air in and out of the body in order to facilitate the exchange of oxygen and carbon dioxide. The respiratory system consists of the nasal passages, pharynx, larynx, trachea, bronchial tubes, lungs, and diaphragm. **Bronchial tubes** branch into **bronchioles**, which end in clusters of alveoli. The **alveoli** are tiny sacs inside the lungs where gas exchange takes place. When the **diaphragm** contracts, the volume of the chest increases, which reduces the pressure in the **lungs**. Then, air is inhaled through the nose or mouth and passes through the pharynx, larynx, trachea, and bronchial tubes into the lungs. When the diaphragm relaxes, the volume in the chest cavity decreases, forcing the air out of the lungs.

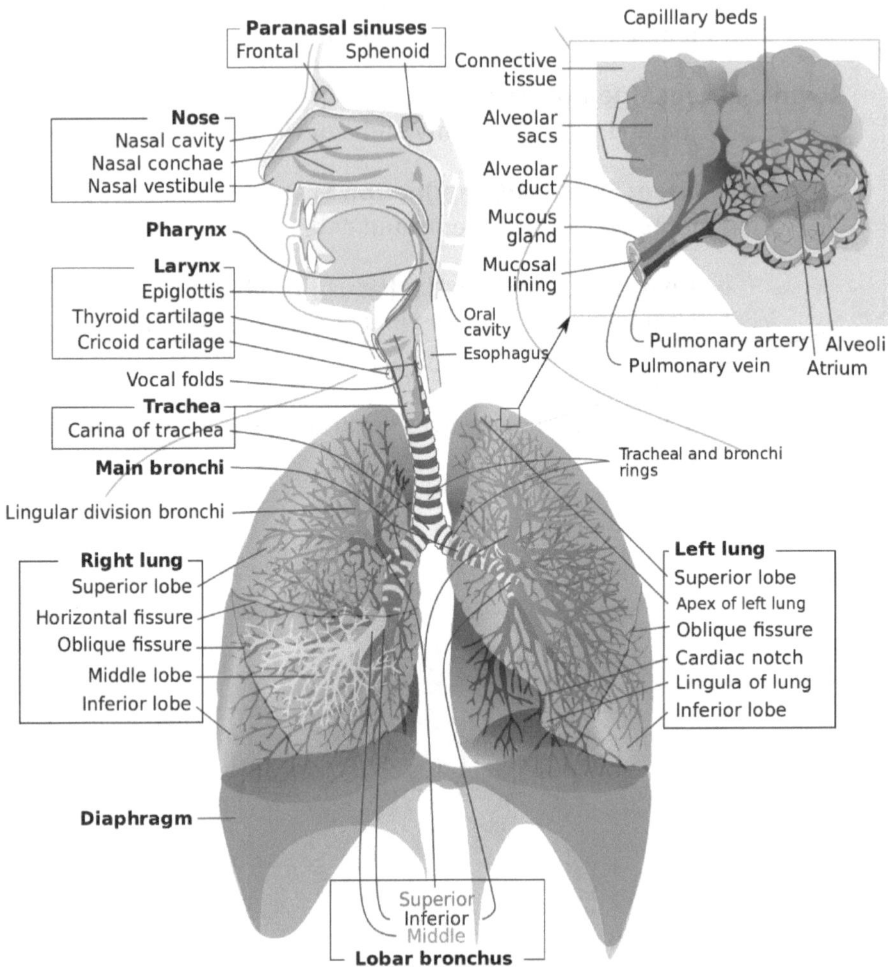

Review Video: Respiratory System
Visit mometrix.com/academy and enter code: 783075

Review Video: What is the Pulmonary Circuit
Visit mometrix.com/academy and enter code: 955608

Reproductive System

The main function of the **reproductive system** is to propagate the species. Most animals reproduce sexually at some point in their life cycle. Typically, this involves the union of a sperm and egg to produce a zygote. In complex animals, the female reproductive system includes one or more ovaries, which produce the egg cell. The male reproductive system includes one or more testes, which produce the sperm.

Review Video: Reproductive Systems
Visit mometrix.com/academy and enter code: 505450

Internal and External Fertilization

Eggs may be fertilized internally or externally. In **internal fertilization** in mammals, the sperm unites with the egg in the oviduct. In mammals, the zygote begins to divide, and the blastula implants in the uterus. Another step in internal fertilization for birds includes albumen, membranes, and egg shell develops after the egg is fertilized. Reptiles lay amniotic eggs covered by a leathery shell. Amphibians and most fish fertilize eggs **externally**, where both eggs and sperm are released into the water. However, there are some fish that give birth to live young.

Invertebrates

Most invertebrates reproduce sexually. Invertebrates may have separate sexes or be **hermaphroditic**, in which the organisms produce sperm and eggs either at the same time or separately at some time in their life cycle. Many invertebrates such as insects also have complex reproductive systems. Some invertebrates reproduce asexually by budding, fragmentation, or parthenogenesis.

Digestive System

The main function of the **digestive system** is to process the food that is consumed by an organism. This includes mechanical and chemical processing. Depending on the organism, **mechanical processes**, or the physical process of breaking food into smaller pieces, can happen in various ways. Mammals have teeth to chew their food, while many animals such as birds, earthworms, crocodilians, and crustaceans have a gizzard or gizzard-like organ that grinds their food. **Chemical digestion** includes breaking food into simpler nutrients that the body can use for specific processes. While chewing, saliva (which contains special enzymes) is secreted to begin the breakdown of starches. Many animals such as mammals, birds, reptiles, amphibians, and fish have a stomach that stores and absorbs food. Gastric juice containing enzymes and hydrochloric acid is mixed with the food. The intestine or intestines absorb nutrients and reabsorb water from the undigested material. Additionally, many animals have a liver, gallbladder, and pancreas, which aid in digestion of proteins and fats. Undigested wasted are eliminated from the body through an anus or cloaca.

Review Video: Gastrointestinal System
Visit mometrix.com/academy and enter code: 378740

Excretory System

All animals have some type of **excretory system** that has the main function of eliminating metabolic waste and excess substances. In complex animals such as mammals, the excretory system consists of the kidneys, ureters, urinary bladder, and urethra. Urea and other toxic wastes must be eliminated from the body. The kidneys constantly filter the blood and facilitate nutrient reabsorption and waste secretion. Urine passes from the kidneys through the ureters to the urinary bladder where it is stored before it is expelled from the body through the urethra.

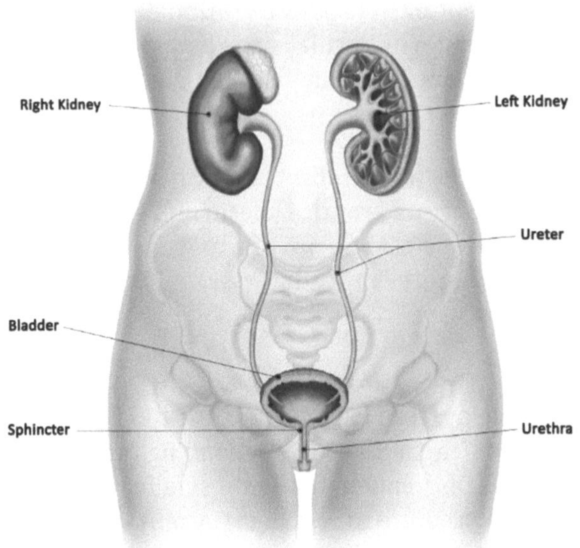

KIDNEYS

The **kidneys** are involved in blood filtration, pH balance, and the reabsorption of nutrients to maintain proper blood volume and ion balance. The **nephron** is the working unit of the kidney. The parts of the nephron include the glomerulus, Bowman's capsule, and loop of Henle. Filtration takes place in the nephron's **glomerulus.** Water and dissolved materials such as glucose and amino acids pass on into the Bowman's capsule. Depending on concentration gradients, water and dissolved materials can pass back into the blood primarily through the proximal convoluted tubule. Reabsorption and water removal occurs in the **loop of Henle** and the conducting duct. Urine and other nitrogenous wastes pass from the kidneys to the bladders and are expelled.

Review Video: Urinary System
Visit mometrix.com/academy and enter code: 601053

NERVOUS SYSTEM

All animals except sponges have a nervous system. The main function of the **nervous system** is to coordinate the activities of the body. The nervous system consists of the brain, spinal cord, peripheral nerves, and sense organs. **Sensory organs** such as the ears, eyes, nose, taste buds, and pressure receptors receive stimuli from the environment and relay that information through nerves and the spinal cord to the brain where the information is processed. The **brain** sends signals through the spinal cord and peripheral nerves to the organs and muscles. The **autonomic nervous system** controls all routine body functions by the sympathetic and parasympathetic divisions. Reflexes, which are also part of the nervous system, may involve only a few nerve cells and bypass the brain when an immediate response is necessary.

Review Video: Autonomic Nervous System
Visit mometrix.com/academy and enter code: 598501

Endocrine System

The **endocrine system** consists of several ductless glands, which secrete hormones directly into the bloodstream. The **pituitary gland** controls the functions of the other glands in the system, regulates skeletal growth, and initiates the development of reproductive organs. The **pineal gland** regulates sleep cycles. The **thyroid gland** regulates metabolism and work with the **parathyroid glands** to help regulate the calcium level in the blood. The **adrenal glands** secrete the emergency hormone epinephrine, stimulate body repairs, and regulate sodium and potassium levels in the blood. The **islets of Langerhans**, located in the pancreas, secrete insulin and glucagon to regulate the level of blood sugar. In females, **ovaries** produce estrogen, which stimulates sexual development, and progesterone, which functions during pregnancy. In males, the **testes** secrete testosterone, which stimulates sexual development and sperm production.

Review Video: Endocrine System
Visit mometrix.com/academy and enter code: 678939

Immune System

The **immune system** in animals defends the body against infection and disease. The immune system can be divided into two broad categories: innate immunity and adaptive immunity. **Innate immunity** includes the skin and mucous membranes, which provide a physical barrier to prevent pathogens from entering the body. Special chemicals including enzymes and proteins in mucus, tears, sweat, and stomach juices destroy pathogens. Numerous white blood cells such as neutrophils and macrophages protect the body from invading pathogens. **Adaptive immunity** involves the body responding to a specific antigen. Typically, B-lymphocytes or B cells produce antibodies against a specific antigen, and T-lymphocytes or T-cells take special roles as helpers, regulators, or killers. Some T-cells function as memory cells.

Review Video: Immune System
Visit mometrix.com/academy and enter code: 622899

Integumentary System

The integumentary system includes skin, hair, nails, sense receptors, sweat glands, and oil glands. The **skin** is a sense organ, provides an exterior barrier against disease, regulates body temperature through perspiration, manufactures chemicals and hormones, and provides a place for nerves from the nervous system and parts of the circulation system to travel through. Skin has three layers: epidermis, dermis, and subcutaneous. The **epidermis** is the thin, outermost, waterproof layer. The

dermis has the sweat glands, oil glands, and hair follicles. The **subcutaneous layer** has connective tissue. Also, this layer has **adipose** (i.e., fat) tissue, nerves, arteries, and veins.

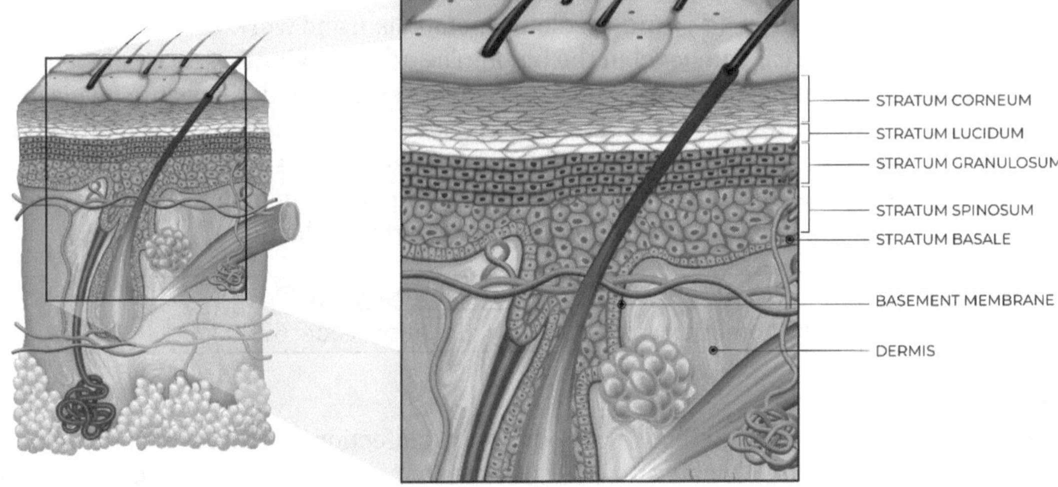

Review Video: Integumentary System
Visit mometrix.com/academy and enter code: 655980

Lymphatic System

The **lymphatic system** is connected to the cardiovascular system through a network of capillaries. The lymphatic system filters out organisms that cause disease, controls the production of disease-fighting antibodies, and produces white blood cells. The lymphatic system also prevents body tissues from swelling by draining fluids from them. Two of the most important areas in this system are the right lymphatic duct and the thoracic duct. The **right lymphatic duct** moves the immunity-bolstering lymph fluid through the top half of the body, while the **thoracic duct** moves lymph throughout the lower half. The spleen, thymus, and lymph nodes all generate and store the chemicals which form lymph and which are essential to protecting the body from disease.

Skeletal System

The skeletal system serves many functions including providing structural support, movement, and protection; producing blood cells; and storing substances such as fat and minerals. The **axial skeleton** transfers the weight from the upper body to the lower appendages. Bones provide attachment points for muscles. The cranium protects the brain. The vertebrae protect the spinal cord. The rib cage protects the heart and lungs. The pelvis protects the reproductive organs. **Joints** including hinge joints, ball-and-socket joints, pivot joints, ellipsoid joints, gliding joints, and saddle joints. The **red marrow** manufactures red and white blood cells. All bone marrow is red at birth, but adults have approximately one-half red bone marrow and one-half yellow bone marrow. Yellow bone marrow stores fat.

Structure of Axial Skeleton and Appendicular Skeleton

The **human skeletal system**, which consists of 206 bones along with numerous tendons, ligaments, and cartilage, is divided into the axial skeleton and the appendicular skeleton.

The **axial skeleton** consists of 80 bones and includes the vertebral column, rib cage, sternum, skull, and hyoid bone. The **vertebral column** consists of 33 vertebrae classified as cervical vertebrae, thoracic vertebrae, lumbar vertebrae, and sacral vertebrae. The **rib cage** includes 12 paired ribs, 10 pairs of true ribs and two pairs of floating ribs, and the **sternum**, which consists of the manubrium, corpus sterni, and xiphoid process. The **skull** includes the cranium and facial bones. The **ossicles** are bones in the middle ear. The **hyoid bone** provides an attachment point for the tongue muscles. The axial skeleton protects vital organs including the brain, heart, and lungs.

The **appendicular skeleton** consists of 126 bones including the pectoral girdle, pelvic girdle, and appendages. The **pectoral girdle** consists of the scapulae (shoulder blades) and clavicles (collarbones). The **pelvic girdle** attaches to the sacrum at the sacroiliac joint. The upper appendages (arms) include the humerus, radius, ulna, carpals, metacarpals, and phalanges. The lower appendages (legs) include the femur, patella, fibula, tibia, tarsals, metatarsals, and phalanges.

The axial skeleton and the appendicular skeleton:

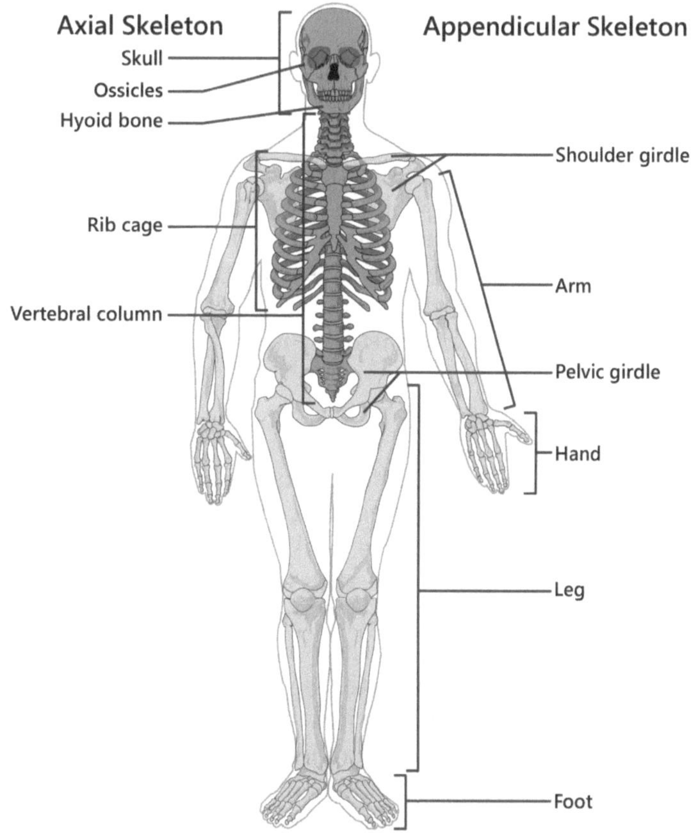

Review Video: Skeletal System
Visit mometrix.com/academy and enter code: 256447

MUSCULAR SYSTEM

Smooth muscle tissues are involuntary muscles that are found in the walls of internal organs such as the stomach, intestines, and blood vessels. Smooth muscle tissues, or **visceral tissue,** is nonstriated. Smooth muscle cells are shorter and wider than skeletal muscle fibers. Smooth muscle tissue is also found in sphincters or valves that control the movement of material through openings throughout the body.

Cardiac muscle tissue is involuntary muscle that is found only in the heart. Like skeletal muscle cells, cardiac muscle cells are also striated.

Skeletal muscles are voluntary muscles that work in pairs to move parts of the skeleton. Skeletal muscles are composed of **muscle fibers** (cells) that are bound together in parallel bundles. Skeletal muscles are also known as **striated muscle** due to their striped histological appearance under a microscope.

Only skeletal muscle interacts with the skeleton to move the body. When they contract, the muscles transmit force to the attached bones. Working together, the muscles and bones act as a system of levers that move around the joints.

Review Video: Muscular System
Visit mometrix.com/academy and enter code: 967216

Major Muscles

The human body has more than 650 skeletal muscles than account for approximately half of a person's weight. Starting with the head and face, the temporalis and masseter move the mandible (lower jaw bone). The orbicularis oculi closes the eye. The orbicularis oris draws the lips together. The sternocleidomastoids move the head. The trapezius moves the shoulder, and the pectoralis major, deltoid, and latissimus dorsi move the upper arm. The biceps brachii and the triceps brachii move the lower arm. The rectus abdominis, external oblique, and erector spine move the trunk. The external and internal obliques elevate and depress the ribs. The gluteus maximus moves the upper leg. The quadriceps femoris, hamstrings, and sartorius move the lower leg. The gastrocnemius and the soleus extend the foot.

Skeletal Muscle Contraction

Skeletal muscles consist of numerous muscle fibers. Each muscle fiber contains a bundle of myofibrils, which are composed of multiple repeating contractile units called sarcomeres. **Myofibrils** contain two protein microfilaments: a thick filament and a thin filament. The **thick filament** is composed of the protein myosin. The **thin filament** is composed of the protein actin. The dark bands (striations) in skeletal muscles are formed when thick and thin filaments overlap. Light bands occur where the thin filament is overlapped. Skeletal muscle attraction occurs when the thin filaments slide over the thick filaments shortening the sarcomere. When an action potential (electrical signal) reaches a muscle fiber, calcium ions are released. According to the sliding filament model of muscle contraction, these calcium ions bind to the myosin and actin, which assists in the binding of the myosin heads of the thick filaments to the actin molecules of the thin filaments. Adenosine triphosphate released from glucose provides the energy necessary for the contraction.

Chapter Quiz

Ready to see how well you retained what you just read? Scan the QR code to go directly to the chapter quiz interface for this study guide. If you're using a computer, simply visit the bonus page at **mometrix.com/bonus948/kaplannursing** and click the Chapter Quizzes link.

Kaplan Nursing Practice Test #1

Want to take this practice test in an online interactive format?
Check out the bonus page, which includes interactive practice questions and much more: **mometrix.com/bonus948/kaplannursing**

Reading Comprehension

Questions 1-4 pertain to the following passage:

It is most likely that you have never had diphtheria. You probably don't even know anyone who has suffered from this disease. In fact, you may not even know what diphtheria is. Similarly, diseases like whooping cough, measles, mumps, and rubella may all be unfamiliar to you. In the nineteenth and early twentieth centuries, these illnesses struck hundreds of thousands of people in the United States each year, mostly children, and tens of thousands of people died. The names of these diseases were frightening household words. Today, they are all but forgotten. That change happened largely because of vaccines.

You probably have been vaccinated against diphtheria. You may even have been exposed to the bacterium that causes it, but the vaccine prepared your body to fight off the disease so quickly that you were unaware of the infection. Vaccines take advantage of your body's natural ability to learn how to combat many disease-causing germs, or microbes. What's more, your body remembers how to protect itself from the microbes it has encountered before. Collectively, the parts of your body that remember and repel microbes are called the immune system. Without the proper functioning of the immune system, the simplest illness—even the common cold—could quickly turn deadly.

On average, your immune system needs more than a week to learn how to fight off an unfamiliar microbe. Sometimes, that isn't enough time. Strong microbes can spread through your body faster than the immune system can fend them off. Your body often gains the upper hand after a few weeks, but in the meantime you are sick. Certain microbes are so virulent that they can overwhelm or escape your natural defenses. In those situations, vaccines can make all the difference.

Traditional vaccines contain either parts of microbes or whole microbes that have been altered so that they don't cause disease. When your immune system confronts these harmless versions of the germs, it quickly clears them from your body. In other words, vaccines trick your immune system in order to teach your body important lessons about how to defeat its opponents.

1. What is the main idea of the passage?

a. The nineteenth and early twentieth centuries were a dark period for medicine.
b. You have probably never had diphtheria.
c. Traditional vaccines contain altered microbes.
d. Vaccines help the immune system function properly.

2. Which statement is *not* a detail from the passage?

a. Vaccines contain microbe parts or altered microbes.
b. The immune system typically needs a week to learn how to fight a new disease.
c. The symptoms of disease do not emerge until the body has learned how to fight the microbe.
d. A hundred years ago, children were at the greatest risk of dying from now-treatable diseases.

3. What is the meaning of the word *virulent* as it is used in the third paragraph?

a. tiny
b. malicious
c. contagious
d. annoying

4. What is the author's primary purpose in writing the essay?

a. to entertain
b. to persuade
c. to inform
d. to analyze

Questions 5-8 pertain to the following passage:

Foodborne illnesses are contracted by eating food or drinking beverages contaminated with bacteria, parasites, or viruses. Harmful chemicals can also cause foodborne illnesses if they have contaminated food during harvesting or processing. Foodborne illnesses can cause symptoms ranging from upset stomach to diarrhea, fever, vomiting, abdominal cramps, and dehydration. Most foodborne infections are undiagnosed and unreported, though the Centers for Disease Control and Prevention estimates that every year about 76 million people in the United States become ill from pathogens in food. About 5,000 of these people die.

Harmful bacteria are the most common cause of foodborne illness. Some bacteria may be present at the point of purchase. Raw foods are the most common source of foodborne illnesses because they are not sterile; examples include raw meat and poultry contaminated during slaughter. Seafood may become contaminated during harvest or processing. One in 10,000 eggs may be contaminated with Salmonella inside the shell. Produce, such as spinach, lettuce, tomatoes, sprouts, and melons, can become contaminated with Salmonella, Shigella, or Escherichia coli (E. coli). Contamination can occur during growing, harvesting, processing, storing, shipping, or final preparation. Sources of produce contamination vary, as these foods are grown in soil and can become contaminated during growth, processing, or distribution. Contamination may also occur during food preparation in a restaurant or a home kitchen. The most common form of contamination from handled foods is the calicivirus, also called the Norwalk-like virus.

When food is cooked and left out for more than two hours at room temperature, bacteria can multiply quickly. Most bacteria don't produce an odor or change in color or texture, so they can be impossible to detect. Freezing food slows or stops bacteria's growth, but does not destroy the bacteria. The microbes can become reactivated when the food is thawed. Refrigeration also can slow the growth of some bacteria. Thorough cooking is required to destroy the bacteria.

5. What is the subject of the passage?

a. foodborne illnesses
b. the dangers of uncooked food
c. bacteria
d. proper food preparation

6. Which statement is *not* a detail from the passage?

a. Every year, more than 70 million Americans contract some form of foodborne illness.
b. Once food is cooked, it cannot cause illness.
c. Refrigeration can slow the growth of some bacteria.
d. The most common form of contamination in handled foods is calicivirus.

7. What is the meaning of the word *pathogens* as it is used in the first paragraph?

a. diseases
b. vaccines
c. disease-causing substances
d. foods

8. What is the meaning of the word *sterile* as it is used in the second paragraph?

a. free of bacteria
b. healthy
c. delicious
d. impotent

Questions 9-12 pertain to the following passage:

There are a number of health problems related to bleeding in the esophagus and stomach. Stomach acid can cause inflammation and bleeding at the lower end of the esophagus. This condition, usually associated with the symptom of heartburn, is called esophagitis, or inflammation of the esophagus. Sometimes a muscle between the esophagus and stomach fails to close properly and allows the return of food and stomach juices into the esophagus, which can lead to esophagitis. In another unrelated condition, enlarged veins (varices) at the lower end of the esophagus rupture and bleed massively. Cirrhosis of the liver is the most common cause of esophageal varices. Esophageal bleeding can be caused by a tear in the lining of the esophagus (Mallory-Weiss syndrome). Mallory-Weiss syndrome usually results from vomiting, but may also be caused by increased pressure in the abdomen from coughing, hiatal hernia, or childbirth. Esophageal cancer can cause bleeding.

The stomach is a frequent site of bleeding. Infections with Helicobacter pylori (H. pylori), alcohol, aspirin, aspirin-containing medicines, and various other medicines (such as nonsteroidal anti-inflammatory drugs [NSAIDs]—particularly those used for arthritis) can cause stomach ulcers or inflammation (gastritis). The stomach is often the site of ulcer disease. Acute or chronic ulcers may enlarge and erode through a blood vessel, causing bleeding. Also, patients suffering from burns, shock, head injuries, cancer, or those who have undergone extensive surgery may develop stress ulcers. Bleeding can also occur from benign tumors or cancer of the stomach, although these disorders usually do not cause massive bleeding.

9. What is the main idea of the passage?

a. The digestive system is complex.
b. Of all the digestive organs, the stomach is the most prone to bleeding.
c. Both the esophagus and the stomach are subject to bleeding problems.
d. Esophagitis afflicts the young and old alike.

10. Which statement is *not* a detail from the passage?

a. Alcohol can cause stomach bleeding.
b. Ulcer disease rarely occurs in the stomach.
c. Benign tumors rarely result in massive bleeding.
d. Childbirth is one cause of Mallory-Weiss syndrome.

11. What is the meaning of the word *rupture* as it is used in the first paragraph?

a. tear
b. collapse
c. implode
d. detach

12. What is the meaning of the word *erode* as it is used in the second paragraph?

a. avoid
b. divorce
c. contain
d. wear away

Questions 13-16 pertain to the following passage:

We met Kathy Blake while she was taking a stroll in the park . . . by herself. What's so striking about this is that Kathy is completely blind, and she has been for more than 30 years.

The diagnosis from her doctor was retinitis pigmentosa, or RP. It's an incurable genetic disease that leads to progressive visual loss. Photoreceptive cells in the retina slowly start to die, leaving the patient visually impaired.

"Life was great the year before I was diagnosed," Kathy said. "I had just started a new job; I just bought my first new car. I had just started dating my now-husband. Life was good. The doctor had told me that there was some good news and some bad news. 'The bad news is you are going to lose your vision; the good news is we don't think you are going to go totally blind.' Unfortunately, I did lose all my vision within about 15 years."

Two years ago, Kathy got a glimmer of hope. She heard about an artificial retina being developed in Los Angeles. It was experimental, but Kathy was the perfect candidate.

Dr. Mark Humayun is a retinal surgeon and biomedical engineer. "A good candidate for the artificial retina device is a person who is blind because of retinal blindness," he said. "They've lost the rods and cones, the light-sensing cells of the eye, but the rest of the circuitry is relatively intact. In the simplest rendition, this device basically takes a blind person and hooks them up to a camera."

It may sound like the stuff of science fiction . . . and just a few years ago it was. A camera is built into a pair of glasses, sending radio signals to a tiny chip in the back of the retina. The chip, small enough to fit on a fingertip, is implanted surgically and stimulates the nerves that lead to the vision center of the brain. Kathy is one of twenty patients who have undergone surgery and use the device.

It has been about two years since the surgery, and Kathy still comes in for weekly testing at the University of Southern California's medical campus. She scans back and forth with specially made, camera-equipped glasses until she senses objects on a screen and then touches the objects. The low-resolution image from the camera is still enough to make out the black stripes on the screen. Impulses are sent from the camera to the 60 receptors that are on the chip in her retina. So, what is Kathy seeing?

"I see flashes of light that indicate a contrast from light to dark—very similar to a camera flash, probably not quite as bright because it's not hurting my eye at all," she replied.

Humayun underscored what a breakthrough this is and how a patient adjusts. "If you've been blind for 30 or 50 years, (and) all of a sudden you get this device, there is a period of learning," he said. "Your brain needs to learn. And it's literally like seeing a baby crawl—to a child walk—to an adult run."

While hardly perfect, the device works best in bright light or where there is a lot of contrast. Kathy takes the device home. The software that runs the device can be upgraded. So, as the software is upgraded, her vision improves. Recently, she was outside with her husband on a moonlit night and saw something she hadn't seen for a long time.

"I scanned up in the sky (and) I got a big flash, right where the moon was, and pointed it out. I can't even remember how many years ago it's been that I would have ever been able to do that."

This technology has a bright future. The current chip has a resolution of 60 pixels. Humayun says that number could be increased to more than a thousand in the next version.

"I think it will be extremely exciting if they can recognize their loved ones' faces and be able to see what their wife or husband or their grandchildren look like, which they haven't seen," said Humayun.

Kathy dreams of a day when blindness like hers will be a distant memory. "My eye disease is hereditary," she said. "My three daughters happen to be fine, but I want to know that if my grandchildren ever have a problem, they will have something to give them some vision."

13. What is the primary subject of the passage?

a. a new artificial retina
b. Kathy Blake
c. hereditary disease
d. Dr. Mark Humayun

14. What is the meaning of the word *progressive* as it is used in the second paragraph?

a. selective
b. gradually increasing
c. diminishing
d. disabling

15. Which statement is *not* a detail from the passage?

a. The use of an artificial retina requires a special pair of glasses.
b. Retinal blindness is the inability to perceive light.
c. Retinitis pigmentosa is curable.
d. The artificial retina performs best in bright light.

16. What is the author's intention in writing the essay?

a. to persuade
b. to entertain
c. to analyze
d. to inform

Questions 17-22 pertain to the following passage:

The immune system is a network of cells, tissues, and organs that defends the body against attacks by foreign invaders. These invaders are primarily microbes—tiny organisms such as bacteria, parasites, and fungi—that can cause infections. Viruses also cause infections, but are too primitive to be classified as living organisms. The human body provides an ideal environment for many microbes. It is the immune system's job to keep the microbes out or destroy them.

The immune system is amazingly complex. It can recognize and remember millions of different enemies, and it can secrete fluids and cells to wipe out nearly all of them. The secret to its success is an elaborate and dynamic communications network. Millions of cells, organized into sets and subsets, gather and transfer information in response to an infection. Once immune cells receive the alarm, they produce powerful chemicals that help to regulate their own growth and behavior, enlist other immune cells, and direct the new recruits to trouble spots.

Although scientists have learned much about the immune system, they continue to puzzle over how the body destroys invading microbes, infected cells, and tumors without harming healthy tissues. New technologies for identifying individual immune cells are now allowing scientists to determine quickly which targets are triggering an immune response. Improvements in microscopy are permitting the first-ever observations of living B cells, T cells, and other cells as they interact within lymph nodes and other body tissues.

In addition, scientists are rapidly unraveling the genetic blueprints that direct the human immune response, as well as those that dictate the biology of bacteria, viruses, and parasites. The combination of new technology with expanded genetic information will no doubt reveal even more about how the body protects itself from disease.

17. What is the main idea of the passage?

a. Scientists fully understand the immune system.
b. The immune system triggers the production of fluids.
c. The body is under constant invasion by malicious microbes.
d. The immune system protects the body from infection.

18. Which statement is *not* a detail from the passage?

a. Most invaders of the body are microbes.
b. The immune system relies on excellent communication.
c. Viruses are extremely sophisticated.
d. The cells of the immune system are organized.

19. What is the meaning of the word *ideal* as it is used in the first paragraph?

a. thoughtful
b. confined
c. hostile
d. perfect

20. Which statement is *not* a detail from the passage?

a. Scientists can now see T cells.
b. The immune system ignores tumors.
c. The ability of the immune system to fight disease without harming the body remains mysterious.
d. The immune system remembers millions of different invaders.

21. What is the meaning of the word *enlist* as it is used in the second paragraph?

a. call into service
b. write down
c. send away
d. put across

22. What is the author's primary purpose in writing the essay?

a. to persuade
b. to analyze
c. to inform
d. to entertain

Writing

Questions 1-5 are based on the following passage.

[1]In Ruth Campbell's book *Exploring the Titanic*, the events of the famous ship's only journey and sinking are brought to life. [2]The *Titanic* was built in 1912, and it was the largest passenger steamship at the time. [3]On what would be its first and only journey, the ship departed from Southampton in England and were supposed to arrive in New York City. [4]The ship hit an iceberg late at night on April 14, 1912, and sank less than three hours later.

[5]The *Titanic* was designed by some of the best engineers and had the latest technology of the time. [6]The ship was made to carry over 3,500 passengers and crew members, but had only 20 lifeboats. [7]There were not enough lifeboats for all of the people onboard, and as a result, only 706 people survived.

[8]One interesting thing about the *Titanic* is that the ship was divided into classes. [9]The most expensive tickets were first class, and first-class passengers had the biggest and most luxerious rooms. [10]Because of this arrangement the majority of the survivors came from first class. [11]They were able to reach the deck fastest to get a seat on a lifeboat. [12]The third-class rooms were located the farthest below deck, and the majority of the third-class passengers did not survive.

[13]Ruth Campbell's book was very interesting, but also sad, because the story of the *Titanic* is true. [14]However, Campbell ended the book by talking about the positive things that have happened because of this tragedy. [15]Most importantly, passenger ships are now required to carry enough lifeboats for all passengers onboard. [16]The *Titanic* had more passenger compartments than any ship that had been built. [17]It was a good book, and it conveyed a good message: in history, mistakes should teach us lessons to keep us from repeating them.

1. Which sentence contains an error in subject-verb agreement?

a. Sentence 3
b. Sentence 7
c. Sentence 10
d. Sentence 12

2. Which of the following changes corrects an error in punctuation?

a. Remove the comma after *onboard* in sentence 7.
b. Add a comma after *arrangement* in sentence 10.
c. Remove the hyphen between *third* and *class* in sentence 12.
d. Add a comma after *things* in sentence 14.

3. Which of the following sentences interrupts the flow of its paragraph by including off-topic information and should be moved or deleted?

a. Sentence 4
b. Sentence 7
c. Sentence 13
d. Sentence 16

4. Which word in the third paragraph is incorrect?

a. The word *expensive* in sentence 9
b. The word *luxerious* in sentence 9
c. The word *arrangement* in sentence 10
d. The word *passengers* in sentence 12

5. Where should the following sentence be added to the third paragraph?

The first-class rooms were the closest to the ship's deck.

a. After sentence 9
b. After sentence 10
c. After sentence 11
d. After sentence 12

Questions 6-10 are based on the following passage.

[1]Basketball is arguably, one of the most popular and most exciting sports of our time. [2]Behind this fast-paced sport, however, is a rich history. [3]There have been many changes made to the game over the years, but the essence remains the same. [4]From it's humble beginnings in 1891, basketball has grown to have a worldwide following.

[5]One thing that sets the history of basketball apart from other major sports is the fact that it was created by just one man. [6]In 1891, James Naismith, a teacher and Presbyterian minister, needed an indoor game to keep college students at the Springfield, Massachusetts, YMCA Training School busy during long winter days. [7]This need prompted the creation of basketball, which was originally played by tossing a soccer ball into an empty peach basket nailed to the gym wall. [8]There was two teams but only one basket in the original game.

[9]Because of the simplicity of basketball, the game had spread across the nation within 30 years of its invention in Massachusetts. [10]As more teams formed, the need for a league became apparent. [11]On June 6, 1946, the Basketball Association of America (BAA) was formed. [12]The smaller National Basketball League (NBL) formed soon after. [13]The NBA played its first full season in 1949-50 and is still going strong today.

[14]Though much has changed in our world in the last hundred years, the popularity of the sport of basketball has remained strong. [15]From a simple YMCA gym to the multimillion-dollar empire it is today, the appeal of the sport has endured. [16]Although many changes have been made over the years, the essence of basketball has remained constant. [17]Its rich history and simplicity ensure that basketball will always be a popular sport around the world.

6. Which of the following changes corrects an error in punctuation?

a. Remove the comma after *arguably* in sentence 1.
b. Add a comma after *sports* in sentence 5.
c. Add a hyphen between hundred and years in sentence 14.
d. Remove the comma after *years* in sentence 16.

7. Which of the following sentences repeats information from earlier in the passage and should be deleted for redundancy?

a. Sentence 5
b. Sentence 8
c. Sentence 12
d. Sentence 16

8. Which word in the passage is incorrect?

a. The word *it's* in sentence 4
b. The word *prompted* in sentence 7
c. The word *apparent* in sentence 10
d. The word *popularity* in sentence 14

9. Which sentence contains an error in subject-verb agreement?

a. Sentence 3
b. Sentence 7
c. Sentence 8
d. Sentence 16

10. Where should the following sentence be added to the third paragraph?

In 1949, the BAA absorbed the NBL, and the National Basketball Association (NBA) was born.

a. After sentence 10
b. After sentence 11
c. After sentence 12
d. After sentence 13

Questions 11-16 are based on the following passage.

[1]The islands of New Zealand are among the most remote of all the Pacific islands. [2]New Zealand is an archipelago, with two large islands and a number of smaller ones. [3]Its climate is far cooler than the rest of Polynesia. [4]According to Maori legends, it was colonized in the early fifteenth century by a wave of Polynesian voyagers who traveled southward in their canoes and settled on North Island. [5]At this time, New Zealand will already be known to the Polynesians, who had probably first landed there some 400 years earlier.

[6]The Polynesian southward migration was limited by the availability of food. [7]Traditional Polynesian tropical crops such as taro and breadfruit would grow on North Island, but the climate of South Island was too cold for them. [8]Coconuts would not grow on either island. [9]The first settlers were forced to rely on hunting gathering, and fishing. [10]Especially on South Island, most settlements remained close to the sea. [11]These flightless birds were easy prey for the settlers, and within a few centuries they had been hunted to extinction. [12]Fish, shellfish, and the roots of the fern were other important sources of food, but even these began to diminish in quantity as the human population increased. [13]The Maori had few other sources of meat: dogs, smaller birds, and rats. [14]Archaeological evidence show that human flesh was also eaten, and that tribal warfare increased markedly after the moa disappeared.

[15]By far the most important farmed crop in precolonial New Zealand was the sweet potato. [16]This tuber was hearty enough to grow throughout the islands, and could be stored to provide food during the winter months, when other food-gathering activities were difficult. [17]Maori tribes often

lived in encampments called *pa*, which were fortified with earthen embancments and usually located near the best sweet potato farmlands. [18]Sweet potatoes have higher starch content than the crops the Maori grew on their native islands. [19]The availability of the sweet potato made possible a significant increase in the human population and allowed the Maori to grow and thrive in relative peace in New Zealand for centuries.

11. Which of the following changes corrects an error in verb usage?

a. In sentence 5, change *will already be* to *was already.*
b. In sentence 7, change *was too cold* to *would be too cold.*
c. In sentence 12, change *began to diminish* to *began diminishing.*
d. In sentence 16, change *was hearty* to *is hearty.*

12. Which word in the passage is incorrect?

a. The word *voyagers* in sentence 4
b. The word *extinction* in sentence 11
c. The word *Archaeological* in sentence 14
d. The word *embancments* in sentence 17

13. Which sentence contains an error in subject-verb agreement?

a. Sentence 4
b. Sentence 12
c. Sentence 14
d. Sentence 18

14. Which of the following changes corrects an error in punctuation?

a. Remove the comma after *archipelago* in sentence 2.
b. Add a comma after *hunting* in sentence 9.
c. Change the colon after *meat* to a semicolon in sentence 13.
d. Remove the hyphen between *food* and *gathering* in sentence 16.

15. Where should the following sentence be added to the passage?

At the time of the Polynesian incursion, enormous flocks of moa birds had their rookeries on the island shores.

a. After sentence 6
b. After sentence 10
c. After sentence 12
d. After sentence 17

16. Which of the following sentences interrupts the flow of its paragraph by including off-topic information and should be deleted?

a. Sentence 7
b. Sentence 12
c. Sentence 15
d. Sentence 18

Questions 17-21 are based on the following passage.

[1]After Orville and Wilbur Wright flew the first successful airplane in 1903, the age of flying slowly began. [2]Many new pilots learned how to fly in World War I, which the United States joined in 1917. [3]During the war, the American public loved hearing stories, about the daring pilots and their

air fights. [4]After the war ended though, many Americans thought that men and women belonged on the ground and not in the air.

[5]In the years after the war and through the Roaring Twenties, many of America's pilots found themselves without jobs. [6]Some of them gave up flying altogether. [7]Pilot Eddie Rickenbacker, who used to be called America's Ace of Aces, became a car salesman. [8]But other pilots, however, found new and creative things to do with their airplanes.

[9]Pilot Casey Jones used his airplane to help get news across the country. [10]When a big news story broke, Jones flew news photos to newspapers in different cities. [11]Another pilot, Roscoe Turner, traveled around the country with a lion cub in his plane. [12]The cub was the mascot of an oil company, and Turner convinced the company that flying the cub around would be a good advertisement. [13]The Humane Society wasn't very happy about this idea, and they convinced Turner to make sure the lion cub always wore a parachute. [14]In the 1920s, the US Postal Service developed airmail. [15]Prior to this, the post traveled on trains and can take weeks to reach a destination, but transporting the post by airplane allowed that time to be cut dramatically.

[16]Flying was dangerous work in those early days, because the aircraft of the time didn't have sophisticated instruments or much safety equipment. [17]Many pilots had to bale out and use their parachutes when their planes iced up in the cold air or had other trouble. [18]Despite all of the dangers and challenges of early aviation, these brave pioneers continued to make use of their ability to fly to advance the state of human civilization.

17. Which of the following changes corrects an error in verb usage?

a. In sentence 2, change *learned* to *learn.*
b. In sentence 5, change *found* to *founded.*
c. In sentence 9, change *used* to *would have used.*
d. In sentence 15, change *can* to *could.*

18. Which word used in the passage is unnecessary and should be deleted?

a. The word *after* in sentence 1
b. The word *altogether* in sentence 6
c. The word *but* in sentence 8
d. The word *because* in sentence 16

19. Which of the following changes corrects an error in punctuation?

a. Remove the comma after *stories* in sentence 3.
b. Remove the comma after *Aces* in sentence 7.
c. Add a comma after *cub* in sentence 12.
d. Add a comma after *out* in sentence 17.

20. Which of the following sentences could be deleted from the third paragraph without disrupting the flow of the passage?

a. Sentence 10
b. Sentence 12
c. Sentence 13
d. Sentence 15

21. Which word in the passage is incorrect?

a. The word *salesman* in sentence 7
b. The word *broke* in sentence 10
c. The word *mascot* in sentence 12
d. The word *bale* in sentence 17

Mathematics

1. Evaluate the expression $\frac{2a}{3b} + 5a - 7b$ when $a = 21$ and $b = 7$.

a. 86
b. 107
c. 64
d. 58

2. Is 45,064 divisible by 8? Explain why.

a. Yes, because it is even.
b. Yes, because the number formed by the last three digits is divisible by 8.
c. Yes, because it begins with an even digit.
d. No, because the last two digits form an even number.

3. What is the LCM of 6 and 10?

a. 28
b. 30
c. 15
d. 60

4. Billy rides his bicycle 5 miles for each morning that he works his paper route. One morning this week, he rode an extra mile to visit with his grandparents. At the end of the week, he had ridden 21 miles. How many mornings did he deliver papers? Support your answer with an equation.

a. 3 mornings; $6x + 3 = 21$
b. 4 mornings; $21x - 5 = 22$
c. 4 mornings; $5x + 1 = 21$
d. 4 mornings; $6x + 3 = 21$

5. Report all decimal places: 3.7 + 7.289 + 4 =

a. 14.989
b. 5.226
c. 15.0
d. 15.07

6. Nora earns $4 per hour at her waitressing job and today received $29 in tips. From her shift today, she earned a total of $53 from both tips and hourly wages. Write an equation from the information given and determine how many hours Nora worked today.

a. $4x + 29 = 53$; Nora worked 6 hours.
b. $29x + 4 = 53$; Nora worked 2 hours.
c. $53x - 29 = 4$; Nora worked 2 hours.
d. $4x - 29 = 53$; Nora worked 9 hours.

7. Karen goes to the grocery store with $40. She buys a carton of milk for $1.85, a loaf of bread for $3.20, and a bunch of bananas for $3.05. How much money does she have left?

a. $30.95
b. $31.90
c. $32.10
d. $34.95

8. Simplify the following expression:

$$7 + 16 - (5 + 6 \times 3) - 10 \times 2$$

a. -42
b. -20
c. 23
d. 20

9. The gas tank in a lawn mower holds up to one liter of gasoline. The gas can used to fill the gas tank of the mower is measured in gallons. Given that there are approximately 3,785 milliliters in a gallon of water, how much of a gallon of gas is needed to fill an empty gas tank of the lawn mower?

a. 0.26 gal
b. 0.20 gal
c. 3.79 gal
d. 1.90 gal

10. Zachary starts his first work shift at 1615. He wants to set an alarm on his phone for 45 minutes before so he knows when to leave for his shift. If his phone uses a 12-hour clock, what time should he set his alarm for?

a. 3:30 PM
b. 4:15 PM
c. 3:30 AM
d. 5:00 AM

11. Aaron worked $2\frac{1}{2}$ hours on Monday, $3\frac{3}{4}$ hours on Tuesday, and $7\frac{2}{3}$ hours on Thursday. How many hours did he work in all?

a. $10\frac{5}{6}$
b. $12\frac{1}{2}$
c. $13\frac{1}{4}$
d. $13\frac{11}{12}$

12. Express the answer in simplest form: Dean has brown, white, and black socks. One-third of his socks are white; one-sixth of his socks are black. What fraction of his socks are brown?

a. $\frac{1}{3}$
b. $\frac{2}{6}$
c. $\frac{1}{2}$
d. $\frac{3}{4}$

13. Express your answer as a mixed number in simplest form: $4\frac{1}{3} \times \frac{2}{7} =$

a. $6\frac{1}{3}$
b. $3\frac{7}{10}$
c. $\frac{8}{21}$
d. $1\frac{5}{21}$

14. Express the answer as a mixed number or fraction in simplest form: $\frac{5}{8} \div \frac{1}{5} =$

a. $\frac{1}{8}$
b. $2\frac{3}{4}$
c. $3\frac{1}{3}$
d. $3\frac{1}{8}$

15. Round to the nearest whole number: Bill got $\frac{7}{9}$ of the answers right on his chemistry test. On a scale of 1 to 100, what numerical grade would he receive?

a. 77
b. 78
c. 79
d. 80

16. Change the fraction to a decimal and round to the hundredths place: $4\frac{3}{7} =$

a. 4.37
b. 4.43
c. 4.56
d. 4.78

17. Change the decimal to the simplest equivalent proper fraction: 0.07 =

a. $\frac{7}{10}$
b. $\frac{0.07}{10}$
c. $\frac{7}{100}$
d. $\frac{70}{100}$

18. Sarah and Elizabeth take a test in their calculus class at school. They are competing for Valedictorian, so they want to compare how they did on their tests. Sarah got $\frac{4}{9}$ questions correct, and Elizabeth, who chose to answer 2 bonus questions, got $\frac{5}{11}$ questions correct. Who did better on the calculus test and how did the girls figure it out?

a. Elizabeth because $\frac{4}{9} > \frac{5}{11}$.
b. Sarah because $\frac{5}{11} < \frac{4}{9}$.
c. Elizabeth because $\frac{4}{9} < \frac{5}{11}$.
d. Sarah because $\frac{4}{9} < \frac{5}{11}$.

19. A bag holds 17 green marbles, 10 blue marbles, and 9 red marbles. Express the ratio of red marbles to total marbles in simplest form.

a. 4 : 36
b. 3 : 12
c. 9 : 36
d. 1 : 4

20. Change the decimal to a percent: 0.64 =

a. 0.64%
b. 64%
c. 6.4%
d. 0.064%

21. The expression $m^3 \times m^8$ is given. Simplify.

a. m^{-5}
b. m^5
c. m^{11}
d. m^{24}

22. Change the percent to a decimal: 126% =

a. 126.0
b. 0.0126
c. 0.126
d. 1.26

23. In a town of 24,821 people, about one fifth of the population is under the age of 20. Of those, approximately three fourths attend local K–12 schools. If the number of students in each grade is about the same, how many first graders likely reside in the town?

a. Fewer than 150
b. Between 150 and 200
c. Between 200 and 250
d. More than 250

24. Round to the nearest percentage point: Gerald made 13 out of the 22 shots he took in the basketball game. What was his shooting percentage?

a. 13%
b. 22%
c. 59%
d. 67%

25. Round to the tenths place: What is 6.4% of 32?

a. 1.8
b. 2.1
c. 2.6
d. 2.0

26. Roger's car gets an average of 25 miles per gallon. If his gas tank holds 16 gallons, about how far can he drive on a full tank?

a. 41 miles
b. 100 miles
c. 320 miles
d. 400 miles

27. Evaluate the expression $8x + 3y - z + 14$ when $x = 2, y = 4$, and $z = 11$.

a. 17
b. 31
c. 63
d. 77

28. Danny is doing a workout program that requires 300 push-ups. Danny wants to divide the push-ups over the span of 5 days. This means that Danny will be completing 20% of the push-ups each day. How many push-ups will Danny do each day?

a. 61 push-ups per day
b. 68 push-ups per day
c. 60 push-ups per day
d. 64 push-ups per day

Science

1. What is the typical result of mitosis in humans?

a. two diploid cells
b. two haploid cells
c. four diploid cells
d. four haploid cells

2. Which of the following is *not* a product of the Krebs cycle?

a. carbon dioxide
b. oxygen
c. adenosine triphosphate (ATP)
d. energy carriers

3. What kind of bond connects sugar and phosphate in DNA?

a. hydrogen
b. ionic
c. covalent
d. overt

4. Which hormone is produced by the pineal gland?

a. insulin
b. testosterone
c. melatonin
d. epinephrine

5. What is the name for a cell that does *not* contain a nucleus?

a. eukaryote
b. bacteria
c. prokaryote
d. cancer

6. What is the longest phase in the life of a cell?

a. prophase
b. interphase
c. anaphase
d. metaphase

7. Which of the following is a protein?

a. cellulose
b. hemoglobin
c. estrogen
d. ATP

8. Which of the following structures is *not* involved in translation?

a. tRNA
b. mRNA
c. ribosome
d. DNA

9. Which of the following is necessary for cell diffusion?

a. water
b. membrane
c. ATP
d. gradient

10. Which part of aerobic respiration uses oxygen?

a. osmosis
b. Krebs cycle
c. glycolysis
d. electron transport system

11. Where is the parathyroid gland located?

a. neck
b. back
c. side
d. brain

12. Which structure of the nervous system carries action potential in the direction of a synapse?

a. cell body
b. axon
c. neuron
d. myelin

13. Which structure controls the hormones secreted by the pituitary gland?

a. hypothalamus
b. adrenal gland
c. testes
d. pancreas

14. Which of the following hormones decreases the concentration of blood glucose?

a. insulin
b. glucagon
c. growth hormone
d. glucocorticoids

15. Which structure in the brain is responsible for arousal and maintenance of consciousness?

a. The midbrain
b. The reticular activating system
c. The diencephalon
d. The limbic system

16. Which layer of the heart contains striated muscle fibers for contraction of the heart?

a. Pericardium
b. Epicardium
c. Endocardium
d. Myocardium

17. Which granulocyte is most likely to be elevated during an allergic response?

a. Neutrophil
b. Monocyte
c. Eosinophil
d. Basophil

18. Cricoid cartilage is found on the:

a. alveoli
b. bronchioles
c. bronchi
d. trachea

19. What is the proper order of the divisions of the small intestine as food passes through the gastrointestinal tract?

a. Ileum, duodenum, jejunum
b. Duodenum, Ileum, jejunum
c. Duodenum, jejunum, ileum
d. Ileum, jejunum, duodenum

20. Which range represents the normal pH of the body fluids?

a. 7.05 to 7.15
b. 7.15 to 7.25
c. 7.25 to 7.35
d. 7.35 to 7.45

Answer Key and Explanations for Test #1

Reading Comprehension

1. D: The main idea of this passage is that vaccines help the immune system function properly. Identifying main ideas is one of the key skills tested on the exam. One of the common traps that many test-takers fall into is assuming that the first sentence of the passage will express the main idea. Although this will be true for some passages, often the author will use the first sentence to attract interest or to make an introductory, but not central, point. On this question, if you assume that the first sentence contains the main idea, you will incorrectly choose answer B. Finding the main idea of a passage requires patience and thoroughness; you cannot expect to know the main idea until you have read the entire passage. In this case, a diligent reading will show you that answer choices A, B, and C express details from the passage, but only answer choice D is a comprehensive summary of the author's message.

2. C: This passage does not state that the symptoms of disease will not emerge until the body has learned to fight the disease. The reading comprehension section of the exam will include several questions that require you to identify details from a passage. The typical structure of these questions is to ask you to identify the answer choice that contains a detail not included in the passage. This question structure makes your work a little more difficult, because it requires you to confirm that the other three details are in the passage. In this question, the details expressed in answer choices A, B, and D are all explicit in the passage. The passage never states, however, that the symptoms of disease do not emerge until the body has learned how to fight the disease-causing microbe. On the contrary, the passage implies that a person may become quite sick and even die before the body learns to effectively fight the disease.

3. B: In the third paragraph, the word *virulent* means "malicious." The reading comprehension section of the exam will include several questions that require you to define a word as it is used in the passage. Sometimes the word will be one of those used in the vocabulary section of the exam; other times, the word in question will be a slightly difficult word used regularly in academic and professional circles. In some cases, you may already know the basic definition of the word. Nevertheless, you should always go back and look at the way the word is used in the passage. The exam will often include answer choices that are legitimate definitions for the given word, but which do not express how the word is used in the passage. For instance, the word *virulent* could in some circumstances mean contagious. However, since the passage is not talking about transfer of the disease, but the effects of the disease once a person has caught it, malicious is the more appropriate answer.

4. C: The author's primary purpose in writing this essay is to inform. The reading comprehension section of the exam will include a few questions that ask you to determine the purpose of the author. The answer choices are always the same: The author's purpose is to entertain, to persuade, to inform, or to analyze. When an author is *writing to entertain*, he or she is not including a great deal of factual information; instead, the focus is on vivid language and interesting stories. *Writing to persuade* means "trying to convince the reader of something." When a writer is just trying to provide the reader with information, without any particular bias, he or she is *writing to inform*. Finally, *writing to analyze* means to consider a subject already well known to the reader. For instance, if the above passage took an objective look at the pros and cons of various approaches to fighting disease, we would say that the passage was a piece of analysis. Because the purpose of this passage is to present new information to the reader in an objective manner, it is clear that the author's intention is to inform.

5. A: The subject of this passage is foodborne illnesses. Identifying the subject of a passage is similar to identifying the main idea. Do not assume that the first sentence of the passage will declare the subject. Oftentimes, an author will approach his or her subject by first describing some related, familiar subject. In this passage, the author does introduce the subject of the passage in the first sentence. However, it is only by reading the rest of the passage that you can determine the subject. One way to figure out the subject of a passage is to identify the main idea of each paragraph, and then identify the common thread in each.

6. B: This passage never states that cooked food cannot cause illness. Indeed, the first sentence of the third paragraph states that harmful bacteria can be present on cooked food that is left out for two or more hours. This is a direct contradiction of answer choice B. If you can identify an answer choice that is clearly contradicted by the text, you can be sure that it is not one of the ideas advanced by the passage. Sometimes the correct answer to this type of question will be something that is contradicted in the text; on other occasions, the correct answer will be a detail that is not included in the passage at all.

7. C: In the first paragraph, the word *pathogens* means "disease-causing substances." The vocabulary you are asked to identify in the reading comprehension section of the exam will tend to be health related. The makers of the exam are especially interested in your knowledge of the terminology used by doctors and nurses. Some of these words, however, are rarely used in normal conversation, so they may be unfamiliar to you. The best way to determine the meaning of an unfamiliar word is to examine how it is used in context. In the last sentence of the first paragraph, it is clear that pathogens are some substances that cause disease. Note that the pathogens are not diseases themselves; we would not say that an uncooked piece of meat "has a disease," but rather that consuming it "can cause a disease." For this reason, answer choice C is better than answer choice A.

8. A: In the second paragraph, the word *sterile* means "free of bacteria." This question provides a good example of why you should always refer to the word as it is used in the text. The word *sterile* is often used to describe "a person who cannot reproduce." If this definition immediately came to mind when you read the question, you might have mistakenly chosen answer D. However, in this passage the author describes raw foods as *not sterile*, meaning that they contain bacteria. For this reason, answer choice A is the correct response.

9. C: The main idea of the passage is that both the esophagus and the stomach are subject to bleeding problems. The structure of this passage is simple: The first paragraph discusses bleeding disorders of the esophagus, and the second paragraph discusses bleeding disorders of the stomach. Remember that statements can be true, and can even be explicitly stated in the passage, and can yet not be the main idea of the passage. The main idea given in answer choice A is perhaps true, but is too general to be classified as the main idea of the passage.

10. B: The passage never states that ulcer disease rarely occurs in the stomach. On the contrary, in the second paragraph the author states that ulcer disease *can* affect the blood vessels in the stomach. The three other answer choices can be found within the passage. The surest way to answer a question like this is to comb through the passage, looking for each detail in turn. This is a time-consuming process, however, so you may want to follow any initial intuition you have. In other words, if you are suspicious of one of the answer choices, see if you can find it in the passage.

Often you will find that the detail is expressly contradicted by the author, in which case you can be sure that this is the right answer.

11. A: In the first paragraph, the word *rupture* means "tear." All of the answer choices are action verbs that suggest destruction. In order to determine the precise meaning of rupture, then, you must examine its usage in the passage. The author is describing a condition in which damage to a vein causes internal bleeding. Therefore, it does not make sense to say that the vein has *collapsed* or *imploded*, as neither of these verbs suggests a ripping or opening in the side of the vein. Similarly, the word *detach* suggests an action that seems inappropriate for a vein. It seems quite possible, however, for a vein to *tear*: Answer choice A is correct.

12. D: In the second paragraph, the word *erode* means "wear away." Your approach to this question should be the same as for question 11. Take a look at how the word is used in the passage. The author is describing a condition in which ulcers degrade a vein to the point of bleeding. Obviously, it is not appropriate to say that the ulcer has *avoided, divorced*, or *contained* the vein. It *is* sensible, however, to say that the ulcer has *worn away* the vein.

13. A: The primary subject of the passage is a new artificial retina. This question is a little tricky, because the author spends so much time talking about the experience of Kathy Blake. As a reader, however, you have to ask yourself whether Mrs. Blake or the new artificial retina is more essential to the story. Would the author still be interested in the story if a different person had the artificial retina? Probably. Would the author have written about Mrs. Blake if she hadn't gotten the artificial retina? Almost certainly not. Really, the story of Kathy Blake is just a way for the author to make the artificial retina more interesting to the reader. Therefore, the artificial retina is the primary subject of the passage.

14. B: In the second paragraph, the word *progressive* means "gradually increasing." The root of the word is *progress*, which you may know means "advancement toward a goal." With this in mind, you may be reasonably certain that answer choice B is correct. It is never a bad idea to examine the context, however. The author is describing *progressive visual loss*, so you might be tempted to select answer choice C or D, since they both suggest loss or diminution. Remember, however, that the adjective *progressive* is modifying the noun *loss*. Since the *loss* is increasing, the correct answer is B.

15. C: The passage never states that retinitis pigmentosa (RP) is curable. This question may be somewhat confusing, since the passage discusses a new treatment for RP. However, the passage never declares that researchers have come up with a cure for the condition; rather, they have developed a new technology that allows people who suffer from RP to regain some of their vision. This is not the same thing as curing RP. Kathy Blake and others like her still have RP, though they have been assisted by this new technology.

16. D: The author's intention in writing this essay is to inform. You may be tempted to answer that the author's intention is to entertain. Indeed, the author expresses his message through the story of Kathy Blake. This story, however, is not important by itself. It is clearly included as a way of explaining the new camera glasses. If the only thing the reader learned from the passage was the story of Kathy Blake, the author would probably be disappointed. At the same time, the author is not really trying to persuade the reader of anything. There is nothing controversial about these new glasses: Everyone is in favor of them. The mission of the author, then, is simply to inform the reader.

17. D: The main idea of the passage is that the immune system protects the body from infection. The author repeatedly alludes to the complexity and mystery of the immune system, so it cannot be true that scientists fully understand this part of the body. It is true that the immune system triggers the production of fluids, but this description misses the point. Similarly, it is true that the body is under constant invasion by malicious microbes; however, the author is much more interested in the body's response to these microbes. For this reason, the best answer choice is D.

18. C: The passage never states that viruses are extremely sophisticated. In fact, the passage explicitly states the opposite. However, in order to know this, you need to understand the word *primitive*. The passage says that viruses are too primitive, or early in their development, to be classified as living organisms. A primitive organism is simple and undeveloped—exactly the opposite of sophisticated. If you do not know the word *primitive*, you can still answer the question by finding all three of the other answer choices in the passage.

19. D: In the first paragraph, the word *ideal* means "perfect." Do not be confused by the similarity of the word *ideal* to *idea* and mistakenly select answer choice A. Take a look at the context in which the word is used. The author is describing how many millions of microbes can live inside the human body. It would not make sense, then, for the author to be describing the body as a *hostile* environment for microbes. Moreover, whether or not the body is a confined environment would not seem to have much bearing on whether it is good for microbes. Rather, the paragraph suggests that the human body is a perfect environment for microbes.

20. B: The passage never states that the immune system ignores tumors. Indeed, at the beginning of the third paragraph, the author states that scientists remain puzzled by the body's ability to fight tumors. This question is a little tricky, because it is common knowledge that many tumors prove fatal to the human body. However, you should not take this to mean that the body does not at least try to fight tumors. In general, it is best to seek out direct evidence in the text rather than to rely on what you already know. You will have enough time on the exam to fully examine and research each question.

21. A: In the second paragraph, the word *enlist* means "call into service." The use of this word is an example of figurative language, the use of a known image or idea to elucidate an idea that is perhaps unfamiliar to the reader. In this case, the author is describing the efforts of the immune system as if they were a military campaign. The immune system *enlists* other cells, and then directs these *recruits* to areas where they are needed. You are probably familiar with *enlistment* and *recruitment* as they relate to describe military service. The author is trying to draw a parallel between the enlistment of young men and women and the enlistment of immune cells. For this reason, "call into service" is the best definition for *enlist*.

22. C: The author's primary purpose in writing this essay is to inform. As you may have noticed, the essays included in the reading comprehension section of the exam were most often written to inform. This should not be too surprising; after all, the most common intention of any writing on general medical subjects is to provide information rather than to persuade, entertain, or analyze. This does not mean that you can automatically assume that "to inform" will be the answer for every question of this type. However, if you are in doubt, it is probably best to select this answer. In this case, the passage is written in a clear, declarative style with no obvious prejudice on the part of the author. The primary intention of the passage seems to be providing information about the immune system to a general audience.

Writing

1. A: The subject of sentence 3 is *ship*. The sentence has a compound verb, "departed...and were supposed to arrive..." The second part of the compound verb should read "was supposed to arrive" to match the singular subject.

2. B: Sentence 10 begins with the introductory phrase "Because of this arrangement," which should be set off from the rest of the sentence with a comma.

3. D: Sentence 16 contains information about the design of the *Titanic* and should either be moved to paragraph 2, where it would fit better topically, or be deleted from the passage altogether.

4. B: In sentence 9, this word should be spelled *luxurious*. All the other words are spelled and used correctly.

5. A: Note that sentence 10 begins with the transitional phrase "Because of this arrangement." None of the information given in sentence 9 provides a reason for the survivors being primarily first-class passengers. The sentence that is to be inserted, however, does provide an explanation.

6. A: The comma placed after *arguably* in sentence 1 is not called for here. It unnecessarily interrupts the flow of the sentence.

7. D: Sentence 16 expresses exactly the same thought as sentence 3 from the first paragraph. It does not provide any new information and is not necessary for the conclusion of the passage. It should be removed.

8. A: In sentence 4, the possessive pronoun *its* should be used instead of the contraction *it's*. All the other words are spelled and used correctly.

9. C: The verb *was* must be plural to match its closest subject, *teams*.

10. C: Sentences 11 and 12 introduce the BAA and the NBL, but not the NBA. Sentence 13 discusses the inaugural season of the NBA without discussing its origin. Placing the proposed sentence, which explains how the NBA was formed by a merger from the BAA and NBL, after sentence 12 is the most logical option.

11. A: In sentence 5, the verb phrase *will already be* describes a situation that is to exist in the future, but the sentence is discussing something that already exists: the Polynesians' awareness of New Zealand.

12. D: In sentence 17, this word should be spelled *embankments*. All the other words are spelled and used correctly.

13. C: In sentence 14, the subject *evidence* is currently paired with the plural verb *show*. While it is technically uncountable, it should be treated as singular and needs to be paired with a singular verb, such as *shows*.

14. B: Sentence 9 provides a list of activities used by the settlers to acquire food. Items in this list must be separated by commas.

15. B: Sentence 11 begins by referring to "These flightless birds." Sentence 10 does not mention any birds, so placing the proposed sentence (which describes flocks of birds) between these two sentences is ideal.

16. D: The focus of the final paragraph is how the sweet potato allowed the Maori to produce enough food to survive without fighting one another for the limited resources. Sentence 18 interjects an unnecessary piece of information about the nutritional composition of the sweet potato, which interrupts the flow of the paragraph and distracts from its purpose.

17. D: In sentence 15, the subject *post* has a compound verb: "traveled...and can take..." Both verbs need to use the past tense because the action occurs in the past, so *can* should be changed to *could.*

18. C: Sentence 8 does introduce information that is in contrast with what was stated in the previous sentence, but the sentence currently uses two different transitional words to signal that contrast: *but* and *however.* Only one of these signaling words is necessary.

19. A: The comma after *stories* in sentence 3 is unnecessary and should be removed. None of the other suggested changes would improve the passage.

20. C: The third paragraph consists of three examples of the jobs that pilots were able to find in the years following World War I. Each example is introduced and then clarified or explained more fully. Sentence 13 provides extraneous information about the Humane Society's response to one of those jobs. All the other sentences listed here provide information that is necessary to explain the purpose or context of these jobs.

21. D: In sentence 17, the correct word is *bail.* The phrase *bail out* means to jump out of the plane while it is in the air. As a verb, the word *bale* is primarily used to describe the gathering of hay or other similar material into a tightly wrapped roll (a bale).

Mathematics

1. D: To evaluate the expression, first substitute the given values into the expression.

$$\frac{2(21)}{3(7)} + 5(21) - 7(7)$$

From here, simplify using the order of operations.

$$\frac{42}{21} + 5(21) - 7(7)$$

$$2 + 105 - 49$$

$$107 - 49$$

$$58$$

2. B: A number is divisible by 8 if the number formed by the last three digits is divisible by 8. In this case, the number formed by the last three digits (064) is 64, which is divisible by 8. This means that 45,064 is also divisible by 8.

3. B: For small numbers like 6 and 10, the LCM can be determined by simply listing the multiples of each number and then looking for the lowest multiple that appears in both lists.

Multiples of 6: 6, 12, 18, 24, **30**, ...

Multiples of 10: 10, 20, **30,** ...

Lowest multiple in common: 30

4. C: To write the equation for this problem, first decide what x represents. We want to know how many days Billy worked his paper route this week, so x (the unknown) will represent the number of days he worked. Now, notice that Billy rides 5 miles each time he works the paper route. This number describes the *rate* at which he rides daily, so the equation will have 5 multiplied by x.

$$5x$$

We are told that one day during the week, Billy rides an extra mile. Because of this, the equation will include the term $+1$.

$$5x + 1$$

We also are told that Billy rides a total of 21 miles over the week. This will be the number on the other side of the equation.

$$5x + 1 = 21$$

Now, solve for x. Start by subtracting 1 from both sides.

$$5x + 1 - 1 = 21 - 1$$
$$5x = 20$$

Then, divide both sides by 5.

$$\frac{5x}{5} = \frac{20}{5}$$

$$x = 4$$

Billy worked his paper route four mornings this week.

5. A: To solve this problem, you must know how to add a series of numbers when some of the numbers include decimals. As with addition problems 1 and 2, the most important first step is to set up the proper vertical alignment. This step is even more important when working with decimals. Be sure that all of the decimal points are in alignment; in other words, the 7 in 3.7 should be above the 2 in 7.289. Since the final term, 4, is a whole number, we assume a 0 in the tenths place. Similarly, you may assume zeros in the hundredths and thousandths places, if you prefer to have a digit in every relevant place. Then beginning at the rightmost place value (in this case, the thousandths), add the terms together as you would with whole numbers. The decimal point of the sum should be aligned with the decimal points of the terms.

6. A: To write an equation from the information given, first determine "what is the unknown?" In this case, the unknown is how many hours Nora worked. So x will represent the number of hours.

Since Nora is paid \$4 per hour in wages, part of her pay is calculated by multiplying 4 by x. The rest of her pay comes from tips, which are added on top of her hourly pay. Her total pay per shift can be written as $4x + \text{tips} = \text{total}$.

For today's shift, Nora received \$29 in tips and her total pay was \$53. The equation is then $4x + 29 = 53$.

To solve for x, first subtract 29 from both sides.

$$4x + 29 - 29 = 53 - 29$$
$$4x = 24$$

Now, divide both sides by 4.

$$\frac{4x}{4} = \frac{24}{4}$$

$$x = 6$$

So, Nora worked six hours today.

7. B: To solve this problem, you must know how to solve word problems involving decimal subtraction. In this scenario, Karen starts out with a certain amount of money and spends some of it on groceries. To calculate how much money she has left, simply subtract the money spent from the original figure: 40 – 1.85 – 3.20 – 3.05. There is no reason to include the dollar sign in your calculations, so long as you remember that it exists. You cannot subtract the costs of these items at the same time, so you must either subtract them one by one or add them up and subtract the sum from 40. Either way will generate the right answer.

8. B: Start by calculating the amount in parentheses, completing the multiplication first: $5 + 6 \times 3$, which is $5 + 18$, or 23. Then calculate the product at the end: 10×2, which is 20, and complete the equation:

$$\begin{gathered} 7 + 16 - 23 - 20 \\ 23 - 23 - 20 \\ 0 - 20 \\ -20 \end{gathered}$$

9. A: To convert liters to gallons, first convert milliliters to liters. Converting from one metric unit to another requires moving the decimal point in the given measurement to the left or right to determine the value for the required metric unit. The table below shows the prefixes of some of the more common metric units involving volume.

Prefix	kilo-	hecto-	deka-		deci-	centi-	milli-
Symbol	k	h	da		d	c	m
Unit Measure	10^3	10^2	10^1	$10^0 = 1$	10^{-1}	10^{-2}	10^{-3}

When converting a given metric unit that has a smaller unit of measure than the required metric unit, we can move the decimal point for the number having the smaller metric unit the same number of places to the left that it takes to get to the larger metric unit in the table. Since the milliliter metric unit is three places from the liter metric unit, we can move the decimal point that is at the end of 3,785 mL three places to the left to convert it to liters.

$$3.\underset{\smile}{7}\,\underset{\smile}{8}\,\underset{\smile}{5}. = 3.785$$

So, 3,785 mL = 3.785 L.

Alternatively, we could multiply 3,785 mL by ten to the negative third power to get:

$$3{,}785 \times 10^{-3} = 3{,}785 \times \frac{1}{1{,}000} = \frac{3{,}785}{1{,}000} = 3.785$$

Thus, there are approximately 3.785 liters in one gallon of water so, 3.785 L = 1 gal.

Then, to see how much of a gallon of water is in one liter, divide both sides of the equality above by 3.785.

$$\frac{3.785\text{ L}}{3.785} = \frac{1\text{ gal}}{3.785}$$
$$1\text{ L} = 0.264\text{ gal}$$

To the nearest hundredth of a gallon, a liter of water is 0.26 gallons.

10. A: To convert a 24-hour time to 12-hour time, start by subtracting 1200, if the number is greater than 1200.

$$1615 - 1200 = 0415$$

This number corresponds to the 12-hour time in the afternoon, so Zachary's shift starts at 4:15 PM. Since he wants to set an alarm for 45 minutes before, subtract 45 minutes from 4:15 PM, which is

3:30 PM. Therefore, Zachary should set his alarm for 3:30 PM so he knows when to leave for his shift.

11. D: This problem requires you to understand addition involving mixed numbers. The calculation required by this problem is straightforward: In order to derive the number of hours Aaron worked, add up the three mixed numbers. To make this possible, you will need to find the least common multiple of 2, 4, and 3 so that you can establish a common denominator. The lowest common denominator for this problem is 12. You can either add up the whole numbers separately from the fractions or convert the mixed numbers into improper fractions and add them in that form. Either way will yield the correct answer.

12. C: To solve this problem, you must know how to solve word problems requiring fraction addition and subtraction. You are given the proportions of Dean's socks that are white and black. The best approach to this problem is adding together the two known quantities and subtracting the sum from 1. First you need to find a common denominator for $\frac{1}{3}$ and $\frac{1}{6}$. The lowest common multiple of these two numbers is 6, so convert $\frac{1}{3}$ by multiplying the numerator and denominator by 2. The new equation will be $\frac{2}{6}+\frac{1}{6}=\frac{3}{6}$. This sum is equivalent to $\frac{1}{2}$, meaning that half of Dean's socks are either white or black. The other half, then, are brown. If you need to perform the calculation, however, it will look like this: $\frac{2}{2}-\frac{1}{2}=\frac{1}{2}$.

13. D: To solve this problem, you must know how to multiply mixed numbers and fractions. Unlike fraction addition and subtraction, fraction multiplication does not require a common denominator. However, it is necessary to convert mixed numbers into improper fractions. This is done by multiplying the whole number by the denominator and adding the product to the numerator: in this case, $4 \times 3 + 1 = 13$. So, the problem is now $\frac{13}{3} \times \frac{2}{7}$. Fraction multiplication is performed by multiplying numerator by numerator and denominator by denominator: $\frac{13\times2}{3\times7}=\frac{26}{21}$. This improper fraction can be converted into a mixed number by dividing numerator by denominator, which gives $1\frac{5}{21}$.

14. D: To solve this problem, you must know how to divide fractions. The process of dividing fractions is similar to that of multiplying fractions, except that the second term must first be inverted, or replaced with its reciprocal. Once this is done, the numerator is multiplied by the numerator, and the denominator is multiplied by the denominator. This problem can be solved by multiplying $\frac{5}{8}$ by the reciprocal of $\frac{1}{5}$, which is $\frac{5}{1}$ or 5: $\frac{5\times5}{8\times1}=\frac{25}{8}$. Finally, convert this improper fraction into a mixed number according to the usual procedure.

15. B: To solve this problem, you must know how to convert a fraction into a ratio. In this problem, you are being asked to convert the fraction into a value on a scale from 1 to 100, which is basically like being asked to convert it into a percentage. To do so, divide the numerator by the denominator. The answer will be a repeating seven: 0.777.... Calculate to the thousandths place in order to determine the value. Because the digit in the thousandths place is a 7, you will round up the digit to the left to establish the final answer, 78.

16. B: To solve this problem, you must know how to convert mixed numbers into decimals. Perhaps the easiest way to perform this operation is to convert the mixed number into an improper fraction and then divide the numerator by the denominator. Convert the mixed number into an improper fraction by multiplying the whole number by the denominator and adding the product to the numerator: $4 \times 7 + 3 = 31$, so the improper fraction is $\frac{31}{7}$. Next divide 31 by 7, according to the same procedure used in problems 7 and 8. Remember that when you have to add 0 to 31 in order to continue your calculations, you must put a decimal point directly above in the quotient. Also, since the problem asks you to round to the hundredths place, you must solve the problem to the nearest thousandth.

17. C: To solve this problem, you must know how to convert decimals into fractions. Remember that all of the numbers to the right of a decimal point represent values less than one. So, a decimal number such as this will not include any whole numbers when it is converted into a fraction. The 7 is in the hundredths place, so the number is properly expressed as $\frac{7}{100}$. The fraction cannot be simplified because 7 and 100 do not share any factors besides one.

18. C: To determine who did better on the test, compare the two fractions: $\frac{4}{9}$ and $\frac{5}{11}$. The two fractions can be compared by using cross multiplication. When cross multiplying, multiply the numerator of the first fraction by the denominator of the second fraction: $4 \times 11 = 44$. This number corresponds to the first fraction. Then, multiply the denominator of the first fraction by the numerator of the second fraction: $9 \times 5 = 45$. This number corresponds to the second fraction. From here, compare the two numbers: $44 < 45$. This means that the first fraction $\left(\frac{4}{9}\right)$ is less than the second fraction $\left(\frac{5}{11}\right)$: $\frac{4}{9} < \frac{5}{11}$. Since Elizabeth got $\frac{5}{11}$ questions correct on her test, she did better than Sarah.

19. D: There are 9 red marbles and 36 total marbles. This can be expressed as the ratio $9 : 36$. This can be simplified by dividing both 9 and 36 by their greatest common factor (9). The ratio $9 : 36$ becomes $1 : 4$.

20. B: To solve this problem, you must know how to convert a decimal into a percent. A percentage is a number expressed in terms of hundredths. When we say, for instance, that a candidate received 55% of the vote, we mean that she received 55 out of every 100 votes cast. When we say that the sales tax is 6%, we mean that for every 100 cents in the price another 6 cents are added to the final cost. To convert a decimal into a percentage, multiply it by 100 or just shift the decimal point two places to the right. In this case, by moving the decimal point two places to the right you can derive the correct answer, 64%.

21. C: To simplify the expression using the laws of exponents, we use the multiplication rule which states that when two terms with the same base and exponents are being multiplied, we can keep the base and add the exponents. In this case, we keep the base m and add the exponent, $3 + 8$, which equals 11. Therefore, the simplified form of the expression $m^3 \times m^8$ is equal to m^{11}.

22. D: To solve this problem, you must know how to convert percentages into decimals. Remember that a percentage is really just an expression of a value in terms of hundredths. That is, 25% is the same as 25 out of 100. To convert a percentage into a decimal, shift the decimal point two places to the left. In this case, the decimal point is assumed to be after the six in 126%. By shifting the decimal point two places to the left, you find that the equivalent decimal is 1.26.

23. D: The population is approximately 25,000, so one fifth of the population consists of about 5,000 individuals under age 20. Three fourths of 5,000 is 3,750, the approximate number of students in grades K-12. Since there are thirteen grades, there are about 288 students in each grade. So, the number of first graders is likely more than 250.

24. C: To solve this problem, you must know how to convert a fraction into a percentage. Gerald made 13 out of 22 shots, a performance that can also be expressed by the fraction 13/22. To convert this fraction into a percentage, divide the numerator by the denominator: $22\overline{)13}$. Once you derive the initial 5 in the quotient, you can be fairly certain that answer choice C is correct. Whenever possible, try to take these kinds of shortcuts to save yourself some time. Although the exam gives you plenty of time to complete all of the questions, by saving a little time here and there you can give yourself more opportunities to work through the harder problems.

25. D: To solve this problem, you must know how to find equivalencies involving percentages. This problem can be solved with the same strategy used in problem 48. To begin with, set up the following equation: $\frac{6.4}{100} = \frac{x}{32}$. Next cross-multiply: 6.4 × 32 = 100*x*. This produces 204.8 = 100*x*, which is solved for *x* by dividing both sides of the equation by 100. The value of *x* is 2.048, which is rounded to 2.0. Or change the percent to a decimal, 0.064, and multiply by 32 to obtain 2.048 and round to 2.0.

26. D: This problem requires you to understand word problems involving mileage rates and multiplication. The problem states that the car gets an average 25 miles per gallon; in other words, every gallon of fuel powers the car for approximately 25 miles. If the car holds 16 gallons of gas, then, and each of these gallons provides 25 miles of travel, you can set up the following equation: 25 miles/gallon × 16 gallons = 400 miles. Since the first term has gallons in the denominator and the second term has gallons in what would be the numerator (if it were expressed as 16 gallons/1), these units cancel each other out and leave only miles.

27. B: To evaluate this expression, first substitute all the given values into the expression.

$$8(2) + 3(4) - (11) + 14$$

From here, simplify using the order of operations.

$$16 + 12 - 11 + 14$$

$$28 - 11 + 14$$

$$17 + 14$$

$$31$$

28. C: First, figure out what the question is asking. Since we are given the total number of push-ups he wants to do and the percent he will do each day, the question is asking: what number is 20 percent of 300?

Next, turn the question into an algebraic equation.

$$x = 0.2(300)$$

Finally, multiply to solve for x.

$$x = 60$$

Science

1. A: The typical result of mitosis in humans is two diploid cells. *Mitosis* is the division of a body cell into two daughter cells. Each of the two produced cells has the same set of chromosomes as the parent. A diploid cell contains both sets of homologous chromosomes. A haploid cell contains only one set of chromosomes, which means that it only has a single set of genes. For the exam, you will need to know about all the different stages of cell division for both human and plant cells.

2. B: Oxygen is not one of the products of the Krebs cycle. The *Krebs cycle* is the second stage of cellular respiration. In this stage, a sequence of reactions converts pyruvic acid into carbon dioxide. This stage of cellular respiration produces the phosphate compounds that provide most of the energy for the cell. The Krebs cycle is also known as the citric acid cycle or the tricarboxylic acid cycle. The exam may require you to know all stages of cellular respiration: the process in which a plant cell converts carbon dioxide into oxygen.

3. C: The sugar and phosphate in DNA are connected by covalent bonds. A *covalent bond* is formed when atoms share electrons. It is very common for atoms to share pairs of electrons. *Hydrogen* bonds are used in DNA to bind complementary bases together, such as adenine with thymine or guanine with cytosine. An *ionic bond* is created when one or more electrons are transferred between atoms. *Ionic bonds*, also known as *electrovalent bonds*, are formed between ions with opposite charges. There is no such thing as an *overt bond* in chemistry. The exam will require you to understand and have some examples of these different types of bonds.

4. C: *Melatonin* is produced by the pineal gland. One of the primary functions of melatonin is regulation of the circadian cycle, which is the rhythm of sleep and wakefulness. *Insulin* helps regulate the amount of glucose in the blood. Without insulin, the body is unable to convert blood sugar into energy. *Testosterone* is the main hormone produced by the testes; it is responsible for the development of adult male sex characteristics. *Epinephrine*, also known as adrenaline, performs a number of functions: It quickens and strengthens the heartbeat and dilates the bronchioles. Epinephrine is one of the hormones secreted when the body senses danger.

5. C: Prokaryotic cells do not contain a nucleus. A *prokaryote* is simply a single-celled organism without a nucleus. It is difficult to identify the structures of a prokaryotic cell, even with a microscope. These cells are usually shaped like a rod, a sphere, or a spiral. A *eukaryote* is an organism containing cells with nuclei. Bacterial cells are prokaryotes, but since there are other kinds of prokaryotes, *bacteria* cannot be the correct answer to this question. *Cancer* cells are malignant, atypical cells that reproduce to the detriment of the organism in which they are located.

6. B: *Interphase* is the longest phase in the life of a cell. Interphase occurs between cell divisions. *Prophase* is the initial stage of mitosis. It is also the longest stage. During prophase, the chromosomes become visible, and the centrioles divide and position themselves on either side of the nucleus. *Anaphase* is the third phase of mitosis, in which chromosome pairs divide and take up positions on opposing poles. *Metaphase* is the second stage of mitosis. In it, the chromosomes align themselves across the center of the cell.

7. B: *Hemoglobin* is a protein. Proteins contain carbon, nitrogen, oxygen, and hydrogen. These substances are required for the growth and repair of tissue and the formation of enzymes. Hemoglobin is found in red blood cells and contains iron. It is responsible for carrying oxygen from the lungs to the various body tissues. *Adenosine triphosphate* (ATP) is a compound used by living organisms to store and use energy. *Estrogen* is a steroid hormone that stimulates the development of female sex characteristics. *Cellulose* is a complex carbohydrate that composes the better part of the cell wall.

8. D: Deoxyribonucleic acid (*DNA*) is not involved in translation. *Translation* is the process by which messenger RNA (*mRNA*) messages are decoded into polypeptide chains. Transfer RNA (*tRNA*) is a molecule that moves amino acids into the ribosomes during the synthesis of protein. Messenger RNA carries sets of instructions for the conversion of amino acids into proteins from the RNA to the other parts of the cell. *Ribosomes* are the tiny particles in the cell where proteins are put together. Ribosomes are composed of ribonucleic acid (RNA) and protein.

9. A: Water is required for cell diffusion. Diffusion is the movement of molecules from an area of high concentration to an area of lower concentration. This process takes place in the body in a number of different areas. For instance, nutrients diffuse from partially digested food through the walls of the intestine into the bloodstream. Similarly, oxygen that enters the lungs diffuses into the bloodstream through membranes at the end of the alveoli. In all these cases, the body has evolved special membranes that only allow certain materials through.

10. D: The *electron transport system* enacted during aerobic respiration requires oxygen. This is the last component of biological oxidation. *Osmosis* is the movement of fluid from an area of high concentration through a partially permeable membrane to an area of lower concentration. This process usually stops when the concentration is the same on either side of the membrane. *Glycolysis* is the initial step in the release of glucose energy. The *Krebs cycle* is the last phase of the process in which cells convert food into energy. It is during this stage that carbon dioxide is produced and hydrogen is extracted from molecules of carbon.

11. A: The parathyroid gland is located in the neck, directly behind the thyroid gland. It is responsible for the metabolism of calcium. It is part of the endocrine system. When the supply of calcium in blood diminishes to unhealthy levels, the parathyroid gland motivates the secretion of a hormone that encourages the bones to release calcium into the bloodstream. The parathyroid gland also regulates the amount of phosphate in the blood by stimulating the excretion of phosphates in the urine.

12. B: *Axons* carry action potential in the direction of synapses. Axons are the long, fiber-like structures that carry information from neurons. Electrical impulses travel along the body of the axons, some of which are up to a foot long. A *neuron* is a type of cell that is responsible for sending information throughout the body. There are several types of neurons, including muscle neurons, which respond to instructions for movement; sensory neurons, which transmit information about the external world; and interneurons, which relay messages between neurons. *Myelin* is a fat that coats the nerves and ensures the accurate transmission of information in the nervous system.

13. A: The *hypothalamus* controls the hormones secreted by the pituitary gland. This part of the brain maintains the body temperature and helps to control metabolism. The *adrenal glands*, which lie above the kidneys, secrete steroidal hormones, epinephrine, and norepinephrine. The *testes* are the male reproductive glands, responsible for the production of sperm and testosterone. The *pancreas* secretes insulin and a fluid that aids in digestion.

14. A: *Insulin* decreases the concentration of blood glucose. It is produced by the pancreas. *Glucagon* is a hormone produced by the pancreas. Glucagon acts in opposition to insulin, motivating an increase in the levels of blood sugar. *Growth hormone* is secreted by the pituitary gland. It is responsible for the growth of the body, specifically by metabolizing proteins, carbohydrates, and lipids. The *glucocorticoids* are a group of steroid hormones that are produced by the adrenal cortex. The glucocorticoids contribute to the metabolism of carbohydrates, proteins, and fats.

15. B: The reticular activating system (RAS) is primarily responsible for the arousal and maintenance of consciousness. The midbrain is a part of the brainstem, which has a crucial role in the regulation of autonomic functions like breathing and heart rate. The diencephalon consists of the hypothalamus and thalamus in the middle part of the brain between the cerebrum and midbrain. It plays a huge role in regulating and coordinating sensory information and hormonal secretion from the hypothalamus. The limbic system tends to the major instinctual drives like eating, sex, thirst, and aggression.

16. D: The myocardium is the layer of the heart that contains the muscle fibers responsible for contraction (Hint: myo- is the prefix for muscle). The endocardium and epicardium are the inner and outer layers of the heart wall, respectively. The pericardium is the sac in which the heart sits inside the chest cavity.

17. C: Eosinophils are most commonly recruited to deal with allergenic antigens. Monocytes, neutrophils, and basophils also deal with antigens during the immune response, but eosinophils are found to be elevated during an allergic response.

18. D: Cricoid cartilage refers to the thick rings of cartilage that surround the trachea, sitting right above the voice box. The purpose of these thick rings is to serve as additional support and protection for the delicate airway.

19. C: The duodenum is the first segment of the small intestine, connecting to the stomach on one end and to the jejunum on the other. The jejunum sits between the duodenum and the last section of small intestine, the ileum, which then connects to the large intestine.

20. D: There is a very narrow range of normal pH values in the human body, 7.35 to 7.45. Values lower than 7.35 indicate acidosis, and values higher than 7.45 indicate alkalosis. The human body can't function properly if the pH is outside of the normal range.

Kaplan Nursing Practice Tests #2 and #3

To take these additional Kaplan nursing practice tests, visit our bonus page:
mometrix.com/bonus948/kaplannursing

How to Overcome Test Anxiety

Just the thought of taking a test is enough to make most people a little nervous. A test is an important event that can have a long-term impact on your future, so it's important to take it seriously and it's natural to feel anxious about performing well. But just because anxiety is normal, that doesn't mean that it's helpful in test taking, or that you should simply accept it as part of your life. Anxiety can have a variety of effects. These effects can be mild, like making you feel slightly nervous, or severe, like blocking your ability to focus or remember even a simple detail.

If you experience test anxiety—whether severe or mild—it's important to know how to beat it. To discover this, first you need to understand what causes test anxiety.

Causes of Test Anxiety

While we often think of anxiety as an uncontrollable emotional state, it can actually be caused by simple, practical things. One of the most common causes of test anxiety is that a person does not feel adequately prepared for their test. This feeling can be the result of many different issues such as poor study habits or lack of organization, but the most common culprit is time management. Starting to study too late, failing to organize your study time to cover all of the material, or being distracted while you study will mean that you're not well prepared for the test. This may lead to cramming the night before, which will cause you to be physically and mentally exhausted for the test. Poor time management also contributes to feelings of stress, fear, and hopelessness as you realize you are not well prepared but don't know what to do about it.

Other times, test anxiety is not related to your preparation for the test but comes from unresolved fear. This may be a past failure on a test, or poor performance on tests in general. It may come from comparing yourself to others who seem to be performing better or from the stress of living up to expectations. Anxiety may be driven by fears of the future—how failure on this test would affect your educational and career goals. These fears are often completely irrational, but they can still negatively impact your test performance.

Elements of Test Anxiety

As mentioned earlier, test anxiety is considered to be an emotional state, but it has physical and mental components as well. Sometimes you may not even realize that you are suffering from test anxiety until you notice the physical symptoms. These can include trembling hands, rapid heartbeat, sweating, nausea, and tense muscles. Extreme anxiety may lead to fainting or vomiting. Obviously, any of these symptoms can have a negative impact on testing. It is important to recognize them as soon as they begin to occur so that you can address the problem before it damages your performance.

The mental components of test anxiety include trouble focusing and inability to remember learned information. During a test, your mind is on high alert, which can help you recall information and stay focused for an extended period of time. However, anxiety interferes with your mind's natural processes, causing you to blank out, even on the questions you know well. The strain of testing during anxiety makes it difficult to stay focused, especially on a test that may take several hours. Extreme anxiety can take a huge mental toll, making it difficult not only to recall test information but even to understand the test questions or pull your thoughts together.

Effects of Test Anxiety

Test anxiety is like a disease—if left untreated, it will get progressively worse. Anxiety leads to poor performance, and this reinforces the feelings of fear and failure, which in turn lead to poor performances on subsequent tests. It can grow from a mild nervousness to a crippling condition. If allowed to progress, test anxiety can have a big impact on your schooling, and consequently on your future.

Test anxiety can spread to other parts of your life. Anxiety on tests can become anxiety in any stressful situation, and blanking on a test can turn into panicking in a job situation. But fortunately, you don't have to let anxiety rule your testing and determine your grades. There are a number of relatively simple steps you can take to move past anxiety and function normally on a test and in the rest of life.

Physical Steps for Beating Test Anxiety

While test anxiety is a serious problem, the good news is that it can be overcome. It doesn't have to control your ability to think and remember information. While it may take time, you can begin taking steps today to beat anxiety.

Just as your first hint that you may be struggling with anxiety comes from the physical symptoms, the first step to treating it is also physical. Rest is crucial for having a clear, strong mind. If you are tired, it is much easier to give in to anxiety. But if you establish good sleep habits, your body and mind will be ready to perform optimally, without the strain of exhaustion. Additionally, sleeping well helps you to retain information better, so you're more likely to recall the answers when you see the test questions.

Getting good sleep means more than going to bed on time. It's important to allow your brain time to relax. Take study breaks from time to time so it doesn't get overworked, and don't study right before bed. Take time to rest your mind before trying to rest your body, or you may find it difficult to fall asleep.

Along with sleep, other aspects of physical health are important in preparing for a test. Good nutrition is vital for good brain function. Sugary foods and drinks may give a burst of energy but this burst is followed by a crash, both physically and emotionally. Instead, fuel your body with protein and vitamin-rich foods.

Also, drink plenty of water. Dehydration can lead to headaches and exhaustion, especially if your brain is already under stress from the rigors of the test. Particularly if your test is a long one, drink water during the breaks. And if possible, take an energy-boosting snack to eat between sections.

Along with sleep and diet, a third important part of physical health is exercise. Maintaining a steady workout schedule is helpful, but even taking 5-minute study breaks to walk can help get your blood pumping faster and clear your head. Exercise also releases endorphins, which contribute to a positive feeling and can help combat test anxiety.

When you nurture your physical health, you are also contributing to your mental health. If your body is healthy, your mind is much more likely to be healthy as well. So take time to rest, nourish your body with healthy food and water, and get moving as much as possible. Taking these physical steps will make you stronger and more able to take the mental steps necessary to overcome test anxiety.

Mental Steps for Beating Test Anxiety

Working on the mental side of test anxiety can be more challenging, but as with the physical side, there are clear steps you can take to overcome it. As mentioned earlier, test anxiety often stems from lack of preparation, so the obvious solution is to prepare for the test. Effective studying may be the most important weapon you have for beating test anxiety, but you can and should employ several other mental tools to combat fear.

First, boost your confidence by reminding yourself of past success—tests or projects that you aced. If you're putting as much effort into preparing for this test as you did for those, there's no reason you should expect to fail here. Work hard to prepare; then trust your preparation.

Second, surround yourself with encouraging people. It can be helpful to find a study group, but be sure that the people you're around will encourage a positive attitude. If you spend time with others who are anxious or cynical, this will only contribute to your own anxiety. Look for others who are motivated to study hard from a desire to succeed, not from a fear of failure.

Third, reward yourself. A test is physically and mentally tiring, even without anxiety, and it can be helpful to have something to look forward to. Plan an activity following the test, regardless of the outcome, such as going to a movie or getting ice cream.

When you are taking the test, if you find yourself beginning to feel anxious, remind yourself that you know the material. Visualize successfully completing the test. Then take a few deep, relaxing breaths and return to it. Work through the questions carefully but with confidence, knowing that you are capable of succeeding.

Developing a healthy mental approach to test taking will also aid in other areas of life. Test anxiety affects more than just the actual test—it can be damaging to your mental health and even contribute to depression. It's important to beat test anxiety before it becomes a problem for more than testing.

Study Strategy

Being prepared for the test is necessary to combat anxiety, but what does being prepared look like? You may study for hours on end and still not feel prepared. What you need is a strategy for test prep. The next few pages outline our recommended steps to help you plan out and conquer the challenge of preparation.

Step 1: Scope Out the Test

Learn everything you can about the format (multiple choice, essay, etc.) and what will be on the test. Gather any study materials, course outlines, or sample exams that may be available. Not only will this help you to prepare, but knowing what to expect can help to alleviate test anxiety.

Step 2: Map Out the Material

Look through the textbook or study guide and make note of how many chapters or sections it has. Then divide these over the time you have. For example, if a book has 15 chapters and you have five days to study, you need to cover three chapters each day. Even better, if you have the time, leave an extra day at the end for overall review after you have gone through the material in depth.

If time is limited, you may need to prioritize the material. Look through it and make note of which sections you think you already have a good grasp on, and which need review. While you are studying, skim quickly through the familiar sections and take more time on the challenging parts.

Write out your plan so you don't get lost as you go. Having a written plan also helps you feel more in control of the study, so anxiety is less likely to arise from feeling overwhelmed at the amount to cover.

STEP 3: GATHER YOUR TOOLS

Decide what study method works best for you. Do you prefer to highlight in the book as you study and then go back over the highlighted portions? Or do you type out notes of the important information? Or is it helpful to make flashcards that you can carry with you? Assemble the pens, index cards, highlighters, post-it notes, and any other materials you may need so you won't be distracted by getting up to find things while you study.

If you're having a hard time retaining the information or organizing your notes, experiment with different methods. For example, try color-coding by subject with colored pens, highlighters, or post-it notes. If you learn better by hearing, try recording yourself reading your notes so you can listen while in the car, working out, or simply sitting at your desk. Ask a friend to quiz you from your flashcards, or try teaching someone the material to solidify it in your mind.

STEP 4: CREATE YOUR ENVIRONMENT

It's important to avoid distractions while you study. This includes both the obvious distractions like visitors and the subtle distractions like an uncomfortable chair (or a too-comfortable couch that makes you want to fall asleep). Set up the best study environment possible: good lighting and a comfortable work area. If background music helps you focus, you may want to turn it on, but otherwise keep the room quiet. If you are using a computer to take notes, be sure you don't have any other windows open, especially applications like social media, games, or anything else that could distract you. Silence your phone and turn off notifications. Be sure to keep water close by so you stay hydrated while you study (but avoid unhealthy drinks and snacks).

Also, take into account the best time of day to study. Are you freshest first thing in the morning? Try to set aside some time then to work through the material. Is your mind clearer in the afternoon or evening? Schedule your study session then. Another method is to study at the same time of day that you will take the test, so that your brain gets used to working on the material at that time and will be ready to focus at test time.

STEP 5: STUDY!

Once you have done all the study preparation, it's time to settle into the actual studying. Sit down, take a few moments to settle your mind so you can focus, and begin to follow your study plan. Don't give in to distractions or let yourself procrastinate. This is your time to prepare so you'll be ready to fearlessly approach the test. Make the most of the time and stay focused.

Of course, you don't want to burn out. If you study too long you may find that you're not retaining the information very well. Take regular study breaks. For example, taking five minutes out of every hour to walk briskly, breathing deeply and swinging your arms, can help your mind stay fresh.

As you get to the end of each chapter or section, it's a good idea to do a quick review. Remind yourself of what you learned and work on any difficult parts. When you feel that you've mastered the material, move on to the next part. At the end of your study session, briefly skim through your notes again.

But while review is helpful, cramming last minute is NOT. If at all possible, work ahead so that you won't need to fit all your study into the last day. Cramming overloads your brain with more information than it can process and retain, and your tired mind may struggle to recall even previously learned information when it is overwhelmed with last-minute study. Also, the urgent nature of cramming and the stress placed on your brain contribute to anxiety. You'll be more likely to go to the test feeling unprepared and having trouble thinking clearly.

So don't cram, and don't stay up late before the test, even just to review your notes at a leisurely pace. Your brain needs rest more than it needs to go over the information again. In fact, plan to finish your studies by noon or early afternoon the day before the test. Give your brain the rest of the day to relax or focus on other things, and get a good night's sleep. Then you will be fresh for the test and better able to recall what you've studied.

STEP 6: TAKE A PRACTICE TEST

Many courses offer sample tests, either online or in the study materials. This is an excellent resource to check whether you have mastered the material, as well as to prepare for the test format and environment.

Check the test format ahead of time: the number of questions, the type (multiple choice, free response, etc.), and the time limit. Then create a plan for working through them. For example, if you have 30 minutes to take a 60-question test, your limit is 30 seconds per question. Spend less time on the questions you know well so that you can take more time on the difficult ones.

If you have time to take several practice tests, take the first one open book, with no time limit. Work through the questions at your own pace and make sure you fully understand them. Gradually work up to taking a test under test conditions: sit at a desk with all study materials put away and set a timer. Pace yourself to make sure you finish the test with time to spare and go back to check your answers if you have time.

After each test, check your answers. On the questions you missed, be sure you understand why you missed them. Did you misread the question (tests can use tricky wording)? Did you forget the information? Or was it something you hadn't learned? Go back and study any shaky areas that the practice tests reveal.

Taking these tests not only helps with your grade, but also aids in combating test anxiety. If you're already used to the test conditions, you're less likely to worry about it, and working through tests until you're scoring well gives you a confidence boost. Go through the practice tests until you feel comfortable, and then you can go into the test knowing that you're ready for it.

Test Tips

On test day, you should be confident, knowing that you've prepared well and are ready to answer the questions. But aside from preparation, there are several test day strategies you can employ to maximize your performance.

First, as stated before, get a good night's sleep the night before the test (and for several nights before that, if possible). Go into the test with a fresh, alert mind rather than staying up late to study.

Try not to change too much about your normal routine on the day of the test. It's important to eat a nutritious breakfast, but if you normally don't eat breakfast at all, consider eating just a protein bar. If you're a coffee drinker, go ahead and have your normal coffee. Just make sure you time it so that the caffeine doesn't wear off right in the middle of your test. Avoid sugary beverages, and drink enough water to stay hydrated but not so much that you need a restroom break 10 minutes into the